Modern Practical Nursing

This important nursing series, designed specifically for th
Nurse is published as a 'parent' book covering the basic
BASIC NURSING CARE, and a number of smaller h
specialities as the nurse is moved from one disciplin

The following volumes are available;

Parent Book: AN OUTLINE OF BASIC NURSING CARE

Elizabeth M Welsh, RGN, RNT.
Director of Nursing and Midwifery Education, Northern Ireland Counci
Midwives.
Mary Gillespie, RFN, RGN, RCI.
Clinical Instructor, Teaching Division, Glasgow Royal Infirmary and Associated Hospitals.
Catherine Asher, RGN, SCM, RNT.
Senior Nursing Officer, Teaching Division, Glasgow Royal Infirmary and Associated Hospitals.

224 pages 220 illustrations £1.00 net

Volume 1: PAEDIATRIC ORTHOPAEDICS

Mary I Gilchrist, RSCN, RGN, ONC.
Ward Sister, Royal Hospital for Sick Children, Drumchapel Branch, Glasgow.
Noel J. Blockey, FRCS, MChOrth.
Consultant Orthopaedic Surgeon, Royal Hospital for Sick Children, Drumchapel Branch, Glasgow.

112 pages 29 illustrations £0.60 net

Volume 2: THEATRE ROUTINE

Morag H Campbell, RGN, SCM.
Senior Nursing Officer (Theatres & CSSD), Glasgow Royal Infirmary.

160 pages 69 illustrations £0.60 net

Volume 3: PAEDIATRIC SURGERY

Elizabeth D Strathdee, SRN, RSCN.
Ward Sister, Royal Hospital for Sick Children, Glasgow.
D G Young, MB, ChB, FRCS. (Edin), DTM & H.
Senior Lecturer in Paediatric Surgery, The University, Glasgow.
Honorary Consultant Surgeon, Royal Hospital for Sick Children, Glasgow.

96 pages 30 illustrations £0.60 net

Volume 4: DERMATOLOGY

A Keenan, RGN, SCM.
Ward Sister, Glasgow Royal Infirmary.
J O'D Alexander, MB, ChB, FRCP.
Consultant Dermatologist, Glasgow Royal Infirmary.

96 pages 34 black & white, 24 colour illustrations £0.75 net

Volume 5: UROLOGY

Margaret W A Stirling, RGN, SCM.
Ward Sister, Urological Department, Glasgow Royal Infirmary.
Roy Scott, MB, ChB, FRCS. (Glas.), FRCS, (Ed).
Consultant Urologist, Glasgow Royal Infirmary.

80 pages 17 illustrations £0.65 net

Volume 6: PLASTIC SURGERY AND BURNS TREATMENT

Ian T Jackson, MB, ChB, FRCS. (Glas.), FRCS. (Ed).
Consultant Plastic Surgeon, Glasgow & West of Scotland Regional Plastic and Oral Surgery Service, Canniesburn Hospital, Bearsden, Glasgow.
E S Macallan, RGN, SCM, Plastic Surgery Cert.
Former Ward Sister, Glasgow and West of Scotland Regional Plastic and Oral Surgery Service, Canniesburn Hospital, Bearsden, Glasgow. At present a member of the Teaching Staff in the School of Nursing, Glasgow Royal Infirmary and Associated Hospitals.

160 pages — 90 illustrations — £0.60 net

Volume 7: PSYCHIATRY

Emily A Lee, RGN, RMN, RCI. (Edin).
Glasgow Royal Infirmary and Associated Hospitals Teaching Department, Clinical Instructor based at Eastern District Hospital, Glasgow.
A B Sclare, MB, ChB, FRCP. (Glas), FRCP. (Edin), MRCP. (Lond), DPM.
Consultant Psychiatrist, Eastern District Hospital and Glasgow Royal Infirmary, Mackintosh Lecturer in Psychological Medicine, University of Glasgow.

192 pages — £0.60 net

Volume 8: ORTHOPAEDIC SURGERY

Thomas H Norton, MB, ChB, FRCSE.
Consultant Orthopaedic Surgeon to Victoria Infirmary and Philipshill Orthopaedic Hospital, Glasgow.
Judith M Tait, SCM, ONC, RNT.
Senior Nursing Officer, Teaching Division, Glasgow Royal Infirmary School of Nursing.

148 pages — 128 two-colour illustrations — £0.90 net

Volume 9: ADULT MEDICINE

E H R Laird, RGN, SCM, HV Cert.
Unit Nursing Officer, Glasgow Royal Infirmary.
R D Barr, MB, ChB, MRCP.
Registrar, Medical Department, Glasgow Royal Infirmary.

144 pages — 21 illustrations — £0.65 net

Volume 10: ADULT SURGERY

A McWee, RGN, SCM.
Glasgow Royal Infirmary School of Nursing.
M Kennedy Browne, BSc, MD, FRCSE.
Consultant Surgeon, Glasgow Royal Infirmary.

224 pages — 128 illustrations — £1.00 net

Volume 11: MEDICAL PAEDIATRICS

William B Doig, MB, ChB, MRCP, DCH.
Consultant Paediatric Cardiologist, Royal Hospital for Sick Children, Glasgow.
Alison Montford, RSCN, RGN.
Formerly Ward Sister, Royal Hospital for Sick Children, Glasgow.

168 pages — 74 illustrations — £0.95 net

Endocrinology

12

MODERN
PRACTICAL
NURSING
SERIES

Endocrinology

John C Small, SRN, RMN, RNT

Senior Nursing Officer (Education)
Portsmouth Group School of Nursing.

Michael J Clarke-Williams, MA, MB, MRCP(Ed)

Consultant Physician in Geriatric Medicine,
Portsmouth Group Hospitals.

WILLIAM HEINEMANN MEDICAL BOOKS LIMITED
LONDON

First Published 1972

ISBN 0 433 30450 2

Typeset by H Charlesworth & Co Ltd, Huddersfield
Printed in Great Britain by
Redwood Press Limited
Trowbridge, Wiltshire

CONTENTS

Introduction

The endocrine system consists of a number of specialised organs located in different areas of the body. They are called endocrine glands and each produces individual secretions. The products of endocrine glands are called hormones. They pass directly into the blood stream and not through organised ducts, as bile is passed through the biliary apparatus. Because of this characteristic the endocrine gland is also called the ductless gland.

Hormones are complex chemical substances which affect the body by exerting a specific action on organs or groups of cells. Although their action is difficult to define hormones play an active part in metabolism and the normal function of organs and systems. The glands of the endocrine system are:

1 Pituitary or hypophysis
2 Thyroid
3 Parathyroids
4 Islet cells of the pancreas
5 Adrenals
6 Gonads – testis (male), ovary (female)

Metabolic processes of the body are initiated by stimuli of either chemical or nervous origin. The nerve response acts quickly but is of short duration whereas the chemical response acts slowly and is active for a longer period. For many years it was thought that the nervous and endocrine systems functioned independently but research has discovered much evidence showing that the inter-relationship is closer than previously imagined. This particularly involves the hypothalamus which is a part of the nervous system closely associated anatomically with the pituitary gland.

The most important endocrine gland is the pituitary for among its secretions are a number of hormones affecting other glands of the system. These hormones are called 'trophic' hormones because their presence in the circulation stimulates other glands, called 'target' organs,

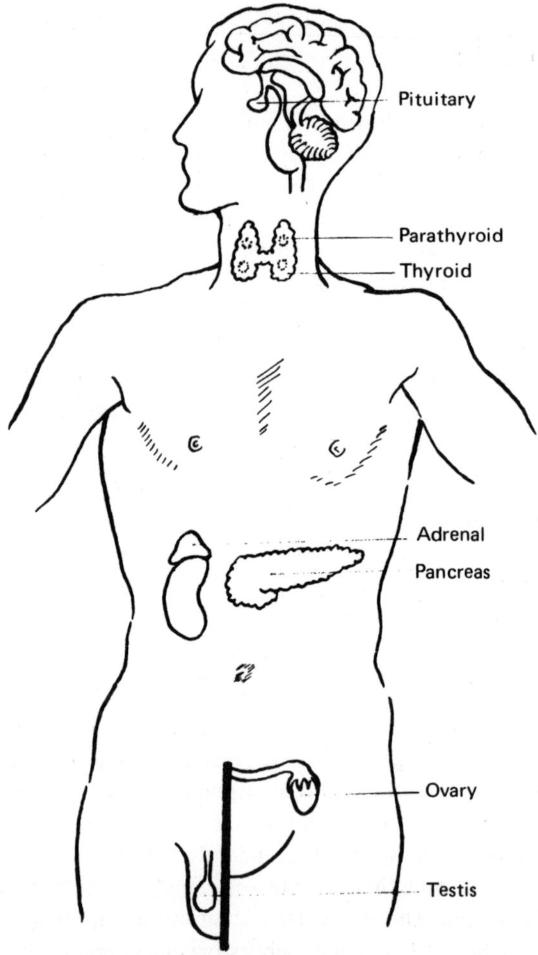

Intro: 1 The endocrine glands

at which they are directed. The concentration of hormone secreted by the target gland in the blood, or the variety of body chemistry created by it, passes back to the pituitary gland. This passage of chemical information is called 'feed back' and allows the pituitary gland to control

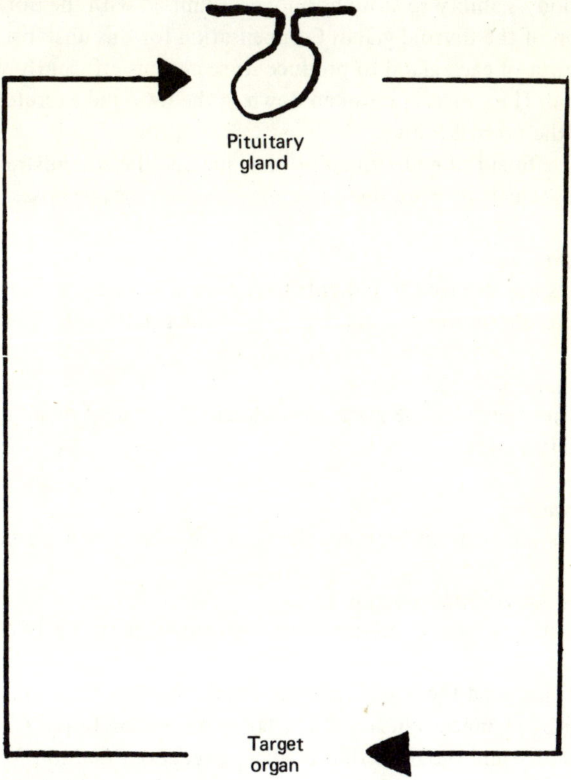

Intro:2 The 'feed back' mechanism

the action of the target gland by regulating the output of trophic hormone. This either increases or reduces the target gland secretion, thus balancing circulating hormones constantly. This pituitary effect is not active on all glands in the system.

Disorders of the endocrine system can be divided into three groups.

1 Oversecretion
2 Undersecretion
3 Secretion of abnormal hormones

The body's ability to store hormones is limited with the notable exception of the thyroid gland. Compensation for this unstable situation is the power of each gland to produce its secretions efficiently when stimulated. Hormones are broken down in the liver and excreted through the normal routes.

The treatment of endocrine disorders include the administration of hormones which are prescribed to create a variety of responses.

1 Replacement

Hormones will be given to patients to replace a deficiency caused by undersecretion or even complete failure of the gland.

2 Stimulation

Trophic hormones can be given to stimulate their target organ in cases of pituitary failure.

3 Retardation

Hormones can be given to retard the effect of abnormal body processes.

4 Reduction of inflammation

Some hormones reduce inflammatory conditions, particularly of allergic origin.

Hormones used therapeutically are obtained either from animal glands or by chemical synthesis. The latter is to be preferred for its greater purity and the reduction of allergic reactions due to protein sensitivity. They can be administered orally, rectally or by injection. Oral hormones are limited to those not inactivated by gastric secretions. Other methods include skin cream, eye drops, snuff and the implantation of pellets for slow absorption.

1

The Pituitary Gland

The pituitary gland, or hypophysis cerebri, is a small pea-shaped organ weighing 0.5gm. It lies at the base of the brain behind and below the crossing optic nerve fibres in the pituitary fossa of the sphenoid bone. This cavity is also called the 'sella turcica' because of its resemblance to the shape of a turkish saddle. Four small protruberances, the clinoid processes, extend over the enclosed gland to complete its protection. The gland is attached to the base of the brain by a short stalk, the infundibulum.

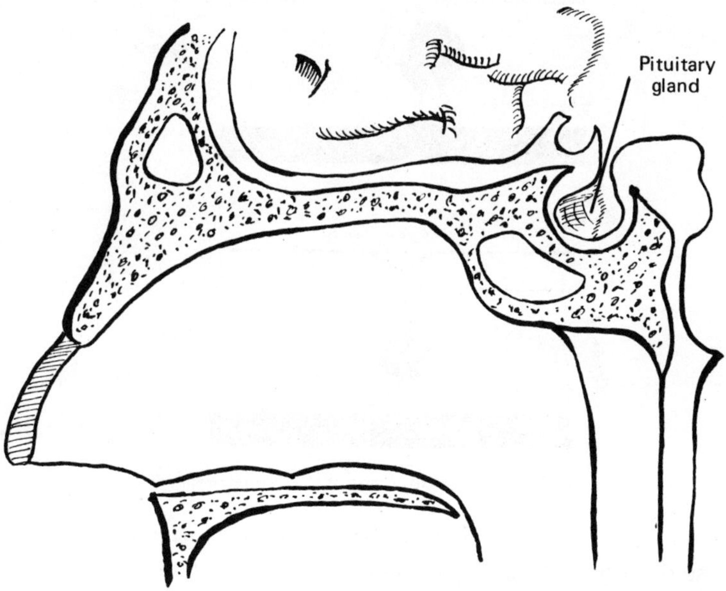

Fig 1:1 Lateral section of skull showing pituitary gland

The pituitary gland is divided into two parts, the anterior and posterior lobes; although anatomically related the two lobes are different in origin, structure and function. In the embryo they are

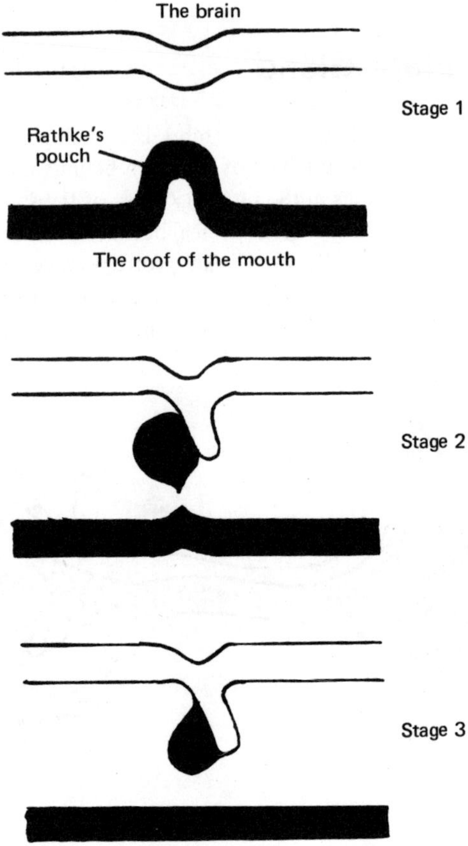

Fig 1:2 Three stages in the development of the pituitary gland

derived from separate sites. The anterior lobe develops from the posterior aspect of the pharynx in the roof of the mouth, called Rathke's pouch. It is glandular in structure and called the adenohypophysis (adeno gland). The posterior lobe develops as a down growth of the brain to which it is attached by the infundubular stalk. It contains a network of nervous tissue and is called the neurohypophysis (neuro nerve).

Like other endocrine glands the pituitary is a very vascular organ, secreting its hormones directly into the circulation. Branches of the internal carotid and posterior communicating arteries – the superior and inferior hypophyseal arteries – supply blood to the infundibular stem and the posterior lobe. Other branches of the internal carotid artery form a capillary network in the hypothalamus leading to a portal system supplying the anterior lobe. The whole complex drains into the hypophyseal veins.

The nerve supply of the pituitary gland is concentrated in the posterior lobe; nerve fibres originating in the hypothalamus descend through the hypophyseal tract and infiltrate the tissues of the lobe. It is thought that secretions of the posterior lobe originate in the hypothalamus and pass down into the gland through small vessels. There is no distinct nerve supply to the anterior lobe although the hypothalamus has a relationship to its function by the passage of hormones via a network of capillaries.

Six hormones are known to be secreted from the adenohypophysis. They are produced from the two types of cells, the acidophils and the basophils. They are trophic in character so that they exert a physiological control over specific distant organs.

1 Somatotrophic or human growth hormone (HGH)
2 Mammotrophin or lactogenic hormone
3 Thyrotrophic or thyroid stimulating hormone (TSH)
4 Corticotrophic or adrenocorticotrophic hormone (ACTH)
5 Follicle stimulating hormone (FSH)
6 Luteinising, or interstitial cell stimulating hormone (LH or ICSH)

Two hormones only are secreted from the neurohypophysis.

1 Vasopressin (Pitressin), or the anti-diuretic hormone (ADH)
2 Oxytocin (Pitocin)

In common with other glands of the system the major disorders are due to an undersecretion or an oversecretion of the hormones.

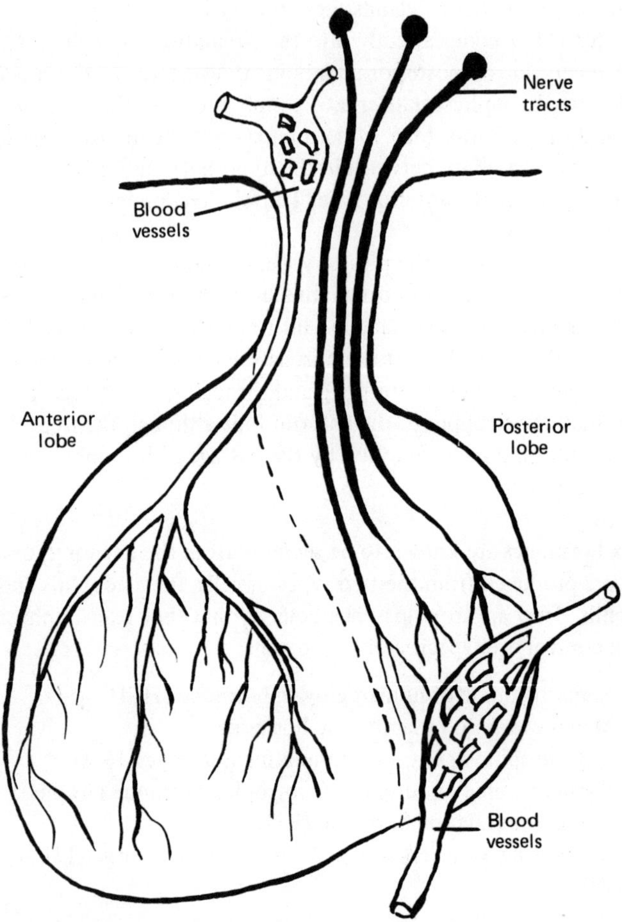

Fig 1:3 Section through the pituitary gland

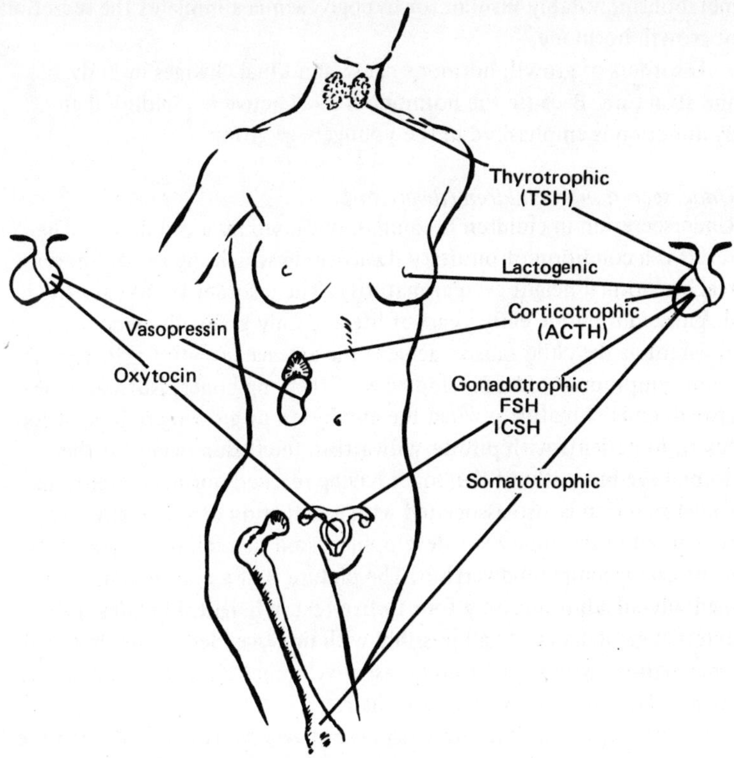

Fig 1:4 Organs affected by pituitary hormones

Adenohypophysis – anterior lobe

Somatotrophic hormone

One function of the anterior lobe is the secretion of a hormone associated with growth. Although its specific action is not fully understood it exerts a powerful effect on the development of body cells, particularly in bone tissue. It is most effective in youth and once growth has stopped it is thought to play a part in repairing and replacing body tissue. Its action is interrelated with other hormones involved in tissue metabolism, notably insulin; for hypoglycaemia stimulates the secretion of growth hormone.

Disorders of growth hormone cause abnormal changes in body size and structure. Because the hormone is most active in childhood any dysfunction is emphasised in the younger age group.

Undersecretion in children (dwarfism)

Undersecretion in children is commonly caused by a cell defect. The result is a condition of pituitary dwarfism in which the subject never reaches normal height even at maturity. The disorder is not easy to diagnose during the early years of life and only gradually becomes apparent as the child fails to achieve the average growth for its age. The main symptom is underdevelopment of the long bones. Normal bone growth ends at maturity when the epiphyses, or growing points, become fused. In patients with pituitary dwarfism the fusion occurs at the normal age but without the bones having reached normal dimensions. Undersecretion is also associated with a reduction of the hormones concerned in secondary sex development and so a failure of sex development can accompany dwarfism. The picture is of a mature person, mentally an adult but only four to five feet in height. In males the external genitalia are small possibly with undescended testes. In females amenorrhoea with little or no breast development is usual. Such patients are also lacking axillary and pubic hair.

Treatment of pituitary dwarfism is not very successful although the use of human growth hormone therapeutically has increased the height of some patients. It is essential that treatment must be started during the early years of life before the growing ends of the bones have fused and natural growth is at its maximum.

Oversecretion in children (gigantism)

In contrast to the retarded growth of long bones in dwarfism, oversecretion causes an excessive growth in the length of the shafts of the long bones. Starting in early childhood this increased growth rate continues until the normal age for fusion of the epiphyses. The patient's height may vary from 6ft 6in to 8ft and his muscles and organs are large in proportion. These patients tend to be strong and appear well developed physically, but the future for the giant is not good. During the years of growing they appear healthy but at maturity they become prone to infection. Death usually occurs before the age of forty, often as the result of an infection that a person of normal size could combat.

The common cause of gigantism is a pituitary tumour. Surgery may be undertaken, particularly if the patient's sight is affected. Implantation of radioactive seeds may reduce the oversecretion of hormone without causing complete hypopituitarism.

Oversecretion in adults (acromegaly)

Oversecretion of growth hormone in adults, after fusion of the bones has occurred, causes acromegaly. The person's height cannot be affected and the excessive growth factor results in bony overgrowth enlarging the mature skeletal structures, particularly the jaw, skull, vertebral bones and the terminal phalanges of the extremities. The jaw becomes abnormally large and tends to jut forward, while the frontal bones of the skull protrude and change the facial appearance. Vertebral bones change shape causing a skeletal deformity. The feet and hands become spade like with massive fingers and palms to the hands. Because this hormone affects tissues other than bone the viscera also enlarge and the abdomen may protrude. Deposits of fat in the subcutaneous layer causes enlargement of the nose, lips and ears, and make the hands appear even larger. The skin and hair become coarse and greasy and the voice deepens due to thickening of the larynx and vocal cords.

The disease progresses slowly and may be unnoticed by the patient for many years. Indeed it may be his friends who first notice that his appearance has changed. The patient may complain of frequent headaches with a deterioration of mental abilities and he may be troubled by muscular weakness and attacks of sweating. The correlation between the hormone of growth and the control of sexual function is demonstrated by a loss of libido and in women amenorrhoea. Other endocrine glands may be involved. A disturbance of insulin secretion causes glycosuria. An affected thyroid increases the metabolic rate and the post-natal patient who is breast feeding her infant may have a prolonged period of lactation.

The most effective form of treatment is insertion of radioactive seeds into the gland, the isotope of choice is Yttrium 90. Hypophysectomy may also be considered as an alternative.

Pituitary tumours

A common cause of pituitary dysfunction is a tumour, which can vary in size and type. They may also cause symptoms of raised intracranial pressure such as headache. Tumours may expand out of the pituitary fossa and press on the optic nerve resulting in disturbances of vision, colour blindness and even complete loss of sight.

The anterior lobe is commonly affected and the tumours are called adenomata being tumours of gland tissue. They are classified by the type of cell involved, that is acidophile, basophile and chromophobe adenomata.

The chromophobe cells are thought to be the precursors of the secretory cells. Sixty per cent of the tumours arise in the chromophobe cells. As they are non-secreting they cause hyposecretion by pressure upon the active cells. Acidophile adenomata are the second largest group, causing acromegaly and gigantism. Basophile adenomata are the rarest type, associated with Cushing's syndrome. Treatment is directed towards control of hormonal secretion and relief of pressure symptoms.

Hypophysectomy

Hypophysectomy is the removal of the pituitary gland. It can be performed directly through the nose or, as is more frequently done, through an incision on the inner angle of the eye.

Pre-operative preparation includes full blood count, estimation of blood sugar and electrolytes, blood pressure recordings and a fluid balance. These tests and observations are used to assess the patient's condition on return from theatre and form a basis on which treatment is established. Skull tomograms are taken to estimate the size and position of the pituitary gland and a chest X-ray taken to ensure the lung fields are clear for anaesthetic. When the pituitary gland is removed it leaves a potential space that must be filled, this is done by the insertion of small pieces of muscle taken from a site on the leg.

The surgeon may request the eyebrow to be shaved if the approach through the inner angle of the eye is made. In male patients the leg is

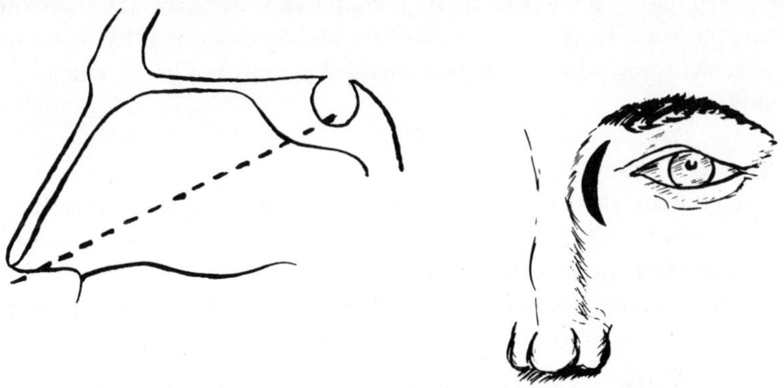

Fig 1:5   Hypophysectomy incisions

shaved ready for the muscle pack to be taken. Drugs prescribed before operation include cortisone by intramuscular injection in readiness for the disturbance of the patient's hormone levels that follows the operation.

Post-operatively careful observation of the blood pressure is necessary and recording must be accurate. Any variations should be reported for the surgeon to review the patient's treatment. An increase in urinary output is caused by the loss of the antidiuretic hormone ADH and will require replacement with pitressin. This is given initially by intramuscular injection of pitressin in tannate oil. Cortisone therapy is continued and an antibiotic may be given to reduce the chance of meningitis developing through the operation site. The nose is packed in theatre and the packing is taken out after seven to ten days, when leaking of cerebro-spinal fluid will be seen. This loss passes down the nose and may continue for days or even weeks, the patient complaining of a running nose and needing constantly to wipe his lip. Electrolyte checks are necessary during the post operative period. They are taken daily and corrective treatment given when needed. Because the operation involves the brain and its coverings the patient may complain of headaches. Analgesics can be given during the acute phase. Sutures are removed from the eye and leg on the seventh day and the patient is discharged after fourteen days if no complications occur.

Hypophysectomy patients are prescribed cortisone acetate, thyroxine and pitressin. These drugs are taken for life, cortisone and thyroxine are in tablet form, pitressin can be prescribed as snuff and taken with an insufflator.

Lactogenic hormone

The pituitary gland's influence on lactation is most apparent when the gland fails for if this occurs lactation ceases. In oversecretion lactation may continue for an abnormally long period.

The pituitary hormone affecting the breast is called prolactin, which has a two-fold function.

1 To interact with ovarian hormones at puberty to promote the growth of breast tissue and the development of secondary sex characteristics.
2 To stimulate lactation after parturition. Milk secretion is maintained by the action of suckling, a reflex which stimulates the production of prolactin.

The hormone is constantly secreted in mature females. After the menopause prolactin ceases to circulate, a change which is attributed to the altered ovarian hormone pattern.

Thyroid stimulating hormone

The pituitary influence on the thyroid gland can be demonstrated when the pituitary gland fails, for such dysfunction is often the precursor to thyroid gland atrophy. The thyroid stimulating hormone controls the function of the gland including the production of thyroxine, its storage in the cells of the gland and its eventual release into the bloodstream.

The release of the trophic hormone is governed by the 'feed back' mechanism in which the blood level of thyroxine is evaluated in the pituitary gland. When the thyroxine level falls 'negative feed back' stimulates the release of TSH in order to increase the output of thyroxine and thus maintain the required level in the blood. There is no efficient method of assessing the level of TSH as the amount in blood is extremely small.

Adrenocorticotrophic hormone
The trophic hormone ACTH controls the function of the adrenal cortex and its effect is to stimulate the secretion of steroids. The adrenal cortex is also controlled by the 'feed back' mechanism for the pituitary gland is sensitive to levels of cortisol (hydrocortisone) which is one of the major steroids secreted by the adrenal cortex.

Gonadotrophic hormones
Two hormones secreted by the adenohypophysis, the gonadotrophins, are concerned with the development and function of the gonads, or sex glands; the hormones are considered separately.

Follicle stimulating hormone
FSH is necessary in both sexes for the development and maturation of the gonads at puberty.

In males FSH initiates the formation of reproductive cells, spermatozoa, and maintains the activity of the testis during reproductive life. This hormone acts directly on testicular structures, particularly the seminiferous tubules in which spermatozoa develop and mature. This gonadotrophic stimulation is activated by the level of testicular secretions carried in the blood. Undersecretion of FSH due to failure of pituitary cells will result in atrophy of the testes and loss of sexual function. Conversely in men with testicular failure, such as after bilateral orchidectomy, where the output of testicular hormone is severely diminished or lost, FSH production rises in an effort to stimulate the gonads.

In females FSH is an important factor in the normal menstrual cycle. At birth each ovary contains many primordial cells. From puberty a number of these cells, or follicles, mature through the influence of the follicle stimulating hormone. As its name suggests FSH initiates menstruation and follicle maturation. During the remainder of the cycle the level of FSH decreases.

Luteinising or interstitial cell stimulating hormone
In males LH or ICSH stimulates secretions of the hormone testosterone from the testis. Its function is the development and maintenance of sex

characteristics in males. In females LH stimulates ovulation and the secretion of oestrogens during the menstrual cycle.

The disorders from the adenohypophysis of secretion of the somatotrophic hormone in adults and children have been discussed. Symptoms of failure in other secretions of the lobe should be considered 'en masse' since the patient demonstrates an involved picture. There are two related disorders to be described. These conditions are caused by complete failure of the adenohypophysis, although they present a similar clinical picture there are two distinct causes.

Simmonds' disease

Simmonds was a German doctor who first described the disease that now bears his name. He connected the patient's signs and symptoms with failure of the pituitary gland caused by trauma, tuberculosis or malignant tumours.

Sheehan's syndrome

Many years later Sheehan demonstrated that one reason for pituitary failure could be described as 'post partum pituitary necrosis'. It is known that the pituitary gland enlarges during pregnancy, this enlargement is natural and after parturition the gland reverts to its normal size. Complications of labour such as severe shock, retention of the placenta and gross haemorrhage may cause failure in the blood supply to the gland, resulting in a state of ischaemia and subsequent death of the tissues.

Whatever the primary cause of anterior lobe failure the effect is shown on the target glands. As the trophic hormones of the gonads, adrenal cortex and thyroid are involved so these organs will fail to function. The result will not be noticed immediately but following the patient's initial disorder their health will slowly deteriorate. At first the patient may display few obvious symptoms although apathy and a lack of interest in themselves may be seen. A complaint of feeling vaguely unwell is also likely. The clinical symptoms can reach their peak in menopausal women.

Certain specific signs can indicate the primary failure, especially in

Sheehan's syndrome where the association of pregnancy is a helpful guide. Because the signs do not appear together it is often difficult for the physician to make an early diagnosis.

1 Failure to lactate could mean prolactin failure, although unsuccessful lactation is clearly not always a positive sign of this disease.
2 Complaints of sensitivity to temperature changes, particularly cold. This is attributed to metabolic disturbances associated with the thyroid gland and undersecretion of thyroxine.
3 Irregular periods or amenorrhoea will develop with failure of the ovaries.
4 Axillary hair is lost and pubic hair becomes scanty, or will not grow again if shaved. Thyroid deficiency will cause the hair of the scalp to recede.

A patient admitted to a medical ward for investigation and diagnosis will present some of these signs on admission. The patient can be male or female, but because of the association with pregnancy the incidence in women is twice as great as that in men. People of any age from early adulthood to sixty years of age can be affected. There is a general wasting of the body which gives the appearance of early senescence. The face has a distinctive waxy pallor and wrinkled, myxoedemic look with creases and marks around the eyes and mouth. The muscular build is flabby and lacks tone. When the nurse bathes the patient she will notice these changes, some of which will be a source of great anxiety, particularly in young women. Routine observations will show that the patient has a slightly subnormal temperature, a slow pulse and a low blood pressure.

The nurse's first thought in caring for this patient should be to relieve the tension and stress which is bound to be present. Her symptoms have been developing for a long time before admission to hospital so the nurse must do all she can to overcome her lethargy and lack of interest. She must try to gain her confidence and co-operation in the investigations and treatment. The patient's attitude will be greatly influenced by the relationship she establishes with the nursing staff. It is not always advisable to enter into detailed discussions about her disorder, but the nurse who shows sympathy, understanding and is a good listener will provide much help and comfort.

From the moment of her admission the patient should be set at ease. She should be given extra privacy when undressing because of the possible embarrassment, and the same consideration is needed when the patient takes a bath. She will be well aware of her deficiencies and may misconstrue the most innocuous comment or remark. It is therefore important that all nurses caring for her understand her problems and are diplomatic and tactful in their approach.

The patient admitted for investigation will be given tests to estimate the performance of the target organs that can be affected by the loss of the trophic hormones.

Adrenal function

A twenty-four hour specimen of urine is tested for steroids lost through the kidneys. It is collected in a large container provided by the laboratory and it is essential that all urine passed during the twenty-four hour period is saved. This must be explained to the patient as she may feel embarrassed and try to avoid using a bedpan every time she wishes to pass urine if she is ambulant and walking in the ward. Many patients are capable of managing their own collection of specimens and this is one way of giving them an interest and involvement in their own treatment. It is important to explain that failure to collect even one specimen could mean repeating the test.

Thyroid function

The following tests can be used to estimate function of the thyroid gland.

1 Basal metabolic rate – the patient's energy requirement when at rest
2 Iodine uptake – to assess the gland's activity
3 Protein bound iodine

Gonad function

Urinalysis will show the level of gonadotrophins excreted, and will substantiate other evidence such as atrophy of the external genitalia and irregular menstruation or amenorrhoea.

Treatment
The aim of the treatment is to replace the hormones produced by the target organs. Three important hormones are considered.

Cortisone. The major hormone of the adrenal cortex is cortisol and this must be replaced in order to regain steroid equilibrium. A suitable dose for the average patient is 12.5mg twice daily.

Thyroxine. The initial doses of thyroxine are small, 0.05mg daily so that metabolism is regulated gradually without straining the heart. The maintenance doses are about 0.2mg per day.

Testosterone and oestrogen. The replacement of sex hormones is important in the younger age group where libido can be restored and genital atrophy prevented. In females the administration of stilboestrol will not stimulate normal menstrual cycles as the levels of both ovarian hormones cannot be corrected to such a critical degree. It does, however, restore libido.

Anorexia nervosa
One disorder which outwardly resembles anterior pituitary failure is anorexia nervosa. This is a condition often found in young women who may initially be overweight, but due to strict weight-reducing diets they develop a morbid hatred of food. Such a patient eventually becomes emaciated, suffers amenorrhoea and appears to be suffering from hypopituitarism. Laboratory investigations show no appreciable loss of hormones and there is no genital atrophy or loss of body hair, indeed there is a fine growth of downy hair over the whole body. Treatment of this condition is largely psychotherapy and a matter of nutrition, for once the patient's weight is restored, her menstrual cycle will recommence.

Hypopituitary coma

The complication of pituitary failure that nurses should understand and look for is pituitary coma. Normal endocrine glands respond automatically to changes in the environment, but in the patient with pituitary failure most of this balance is lost. Because of the lack of trophic hormones the glands are unable to accommodate any serious changes in body function. When the patient is exposed to trauma such as surgery, gross infection or extremes of temperature coma may result. The patient will become drowsy, confused, disorientated and hypothermic, if no treatment is given coma and death will follow. Hypopituitary coma is less likely to occur in patients with a reduced secretion of the gland compared with those with total failure where it may be provoked by stress.

The condition is critical and requires urgent attention. If the patient is already in hospital treatment can be started immediately. In other cases she will be admitted as an emergency. Although her face and extremities appear to be a good colour they will be cold to the touch. Her temperature will be very low and requires a low reading thermometer (75–105°F or 23–40°C) to record it accurately. In spite of this low temperature the patient must not be put into a heated bed but instead should be warmed gradually. Any sudden rise of temperature could create shock to which her body could not adapt. To determine that the rise in the patient's temperature is controlled it should be recorded each quarter of an hour. Any sudden rise should be reported and measures taken to remedy this.

The patient may suffer from 'air hunger' and have difficulty in breathing, so oxygen should be available at the bedside. The level of consciousness should be assessed at regular intervals for this can vary from complete unconsciousness, semi-coma, stupor or drowsiness to complete alertness. Careful and regular observations are needed as the patient's treatment can vary with these changes. A completely unconscious patient is best nursed in the prone position with her head turned to one side, resting on a single pillow. The nurse's principal task is to maintain a clear airway and she will have frequently to remove mucous and other secretions that form in the mouth and air passages. The rule that one should never leave an unconscious patient is important, not only to keep a clear airway but also to prevent her from injuring herself in case she becomes restless. Care of the patient's skin is necessary during this critical period. Modified turning may be used but only under the strict supervision of the sister.

The medical treatment of hypopituitary coma is directed towards the disturbance in normal metabolism. An intravenous infusion is given containing glucose to raise the patient's low blood-sugar level, and sodium to correct the electrolyte imbalance and hydrocortisone. The patient's temperature, pulse and blood pressure are regularly recorded during the acute phase. Such recordings must be accurate as they indicate the progress and effectiveness of the treatment.

Neurohypophysis – posterior lobe

The posterior lobe of the pituitary gland has both a vascular system directly involved with the anterior lobe, and a nervous system connected with the hypothalamus. Any change in body chemistry affecting posterior lobe hormones is thought to react on the hypothalamus, where the hormones are secreted and pass via the small blood vessels alongside the nerve tracts into the posterior lobe to be circulated or stored. Two active hormones are known to be secreted from the posterior lobe.

Vasopressin

Vasopressin, also called pitressin or the antidiuretic hormone (ADH), regulates the reabsorption of water through the kidney tubules according to the proportion of water in the blood. Small clusters of nerve cells (osmoreceptors) in the internal carotid arteries affect the hypothalamus which reacts to high level of water in the blood by reducing the secretion of ADH. Thus the reabsorption of fluid in the proximal tubules of the kidneys is diminished and excretion of fluid is increased. In conditions of dehydration the osmoreceptors stimulate the hypothalamus which increases the secretion of ADH causing greater absorption of water in the kidney. This will continue until a normal water balance is achieved. In normal circumstances ADH is secreted in minute amounts to maintain body water balance. As the name vasopressin suggests it has an effect on smooth muscle contraction but its effect on the blood pressure is insignificant.

Diabetes insipidus

As ADH causes water to be reabsorbed its absence means that the body's ability to take back water from the kidney tubules selectively is lost. The water balance is disrupted and the patient passes large dilute amounts of urine with a correspondingly massive fluid intake to compensate for this. This disorder is called diabetes insipidus, so named to distinguish it from the sugar loaded urine in diabetes mellitus. By comparison with normal urine it is almost pure water. The cause of the disease can be a disorder of the hypothalamus or its tract leading to the posterior lobe.

The disease can affect people of either sex, at any age and it may follow head injury, hypophysectomy or even appear spontaneously. The first sign is a massive thirst particularly for iced water. This thirst never seems satisfied and is accompanied by a large output of urine. The fluid intake needs to be at least equal to the output and if any attempt is made to reduce it the patient will suffer from an intolerable thirst (polydipsia). The patient presents no other direct signs although if a tumour is present headache and disorders of vision may be seen.

The patient's major problem is the difficulty in leading a normal life, being unable to rest for any length of time. During the day he can manage to drink frequently and pass urine when necessary but at night difficulties are caused by this constant need to drink and pass water. The patient cannot rest or take a normal period of uninterrupted sleep and this eventually leads to near exhaustion and collapse.

The patient is admitted to a medical ward for observation and tests to confirm the diagnosis. If he is physically well he will be happier ambulant or sitting in a chair during the day as he is then in a better position to manage the continual problem of drinking and passing urine. To put him at his ease the nurse admitting the patient should ensure that he is given an adequate supply of drinks. It is good practice to nurse the patient in a single room when first admitted to avoid the embarrassment of other patients knowing of his problem, and to allow him greater movement at night without disturbing others in the ward.

Certain specific nursing tasks are necessary. Although it may cause embarrassment to the patient it is imperative that all quantities of fluids passed are charted, as are the fluids taken in drinking. The physician's assessment of the patient's disorder and the subsequent treatment may be based on the intake and output over twenty-four hours. It is important that the patient realises the need for the recordings. He may feel ill at ease passing such large amounts of urine and the temptation to discard them in the toilet will be very strong. It is easier to chart the intake by using a large jug that holds several litres, thus reducing the entries on the fluid chart and avoiding possible mistakes. In twenty-four hours he may pass as much as ten litres of urine of a very low specific gravity, between 1,002–1,006 (normal specific gravity is 1,010–1,030).

The patient's diet must be considered. Although he needs fluids in large amounts it is best to restrict the quantity of tea, alcohol or coffee as these are mildly diuretic and would tend to increase his output. These patients have a voracious appetite and unless the physician requests otherwise food should not be restricted. His appetite will diminish once treatment begins to take effect. The point is again made that to avoid dehydration the fluid taken should at least equal the amount passed.

Confirmation of the diagnosis is necessary before treatment begins. Although this disorder has distinguishing features that would exclude other conditions there are other diseases that present similar symptoms.

Diabetes mellitus

Sugar in the urine of diabetic patients will increase the amount of urine passed. Tests to eliminate diabetes mellitus are necessary.

Hysterical polydipsia

This is a psychiatric disorder of compulsive water drinking. The patient takes abnormally large amounts of fluid, with a subsequent large output of urine. If the intake of fluid is restricted the urine output drops and the patient does not become dehydrated.

Chronic renal disorders

Some renal diseases give rise to increases in urinary output, this is related to the failure of the kidney to concentrate urine. Other distinguishing features of renal disorder would be present to differentiate the diagnosis.

Tests for diabetes insipidus are limited, ADH cannot be estimated in the blood so other methods must be used. A test dose of vasopressin five to fifteen units may be given intramuscularly. In positive cases this will lower the output of urine and raise the specific gravity. Although a useful indicator the pressor effect on the circulation will cause a rise in blood pressure and produce headaches. One test, which unfortunately causes great hardship to the patient, is called the fluid deprivation test. The patient takes no fluids or fruit for twenty-four hours, at the end of this time the specific gravity of the urine is estimated. In confirmed cases the specific gravity will remain at 1,005 to 1,010 while in normal patients it will rise to 1,030.

Treatment
This is directed at replacing the hormone vasopressin. Because gastric secretions destroy the active constituents it cannot be given orally, but there are two alternative methods of administration.

Pitressin can be given by intramuscular injection of vasopressin tannate in oily solution. The effect is short lived and so this is not a suitable method for long-term treatment.

Fortunately pitressin can also be administered in the form of snuff. This is manufactured in small capsules which are perforated with a pin and placed in an insufflator. Each capsule contains approximately thirty units of ADH hormone and insufflation into the nostrils is carried out according to the physician's directions.

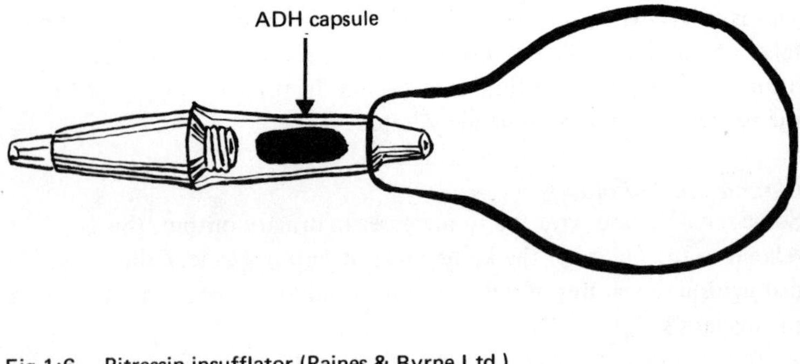

Fig 1:6 Pitressin insufflator (Paines & Byrne Ltd.)

Oxytocin

The hormone oxytocin, or pitocin, has two functions. It stimulates contraction of smooth muscle, particularly the uterus at term, and it is involved with lactation and the movement of milk in the breast.

Oxytocin affects the uterus at parturition. The non-gravid uterus is not affected and during pregnancy progesterone restricts the action of oxytocin until the onset of labour. Because of its contracting effect extracts of oxytocin have found a useful place in obstetrics. When it is necessary to induce labour, as in premature rupture of the membranes or toxaemia, oxytocin can be given. It is also used therapeutically to control post-partum haemorrhage.

Oxytocin can be given by subcutaneous or intramuscular injection, when doses of 0.5 to 1.0ml are used. The dose is carefully assessed as the drug produces powerful contractions. It can also be given orally as tablets to be absorbed slowly when placed between the cheek and the molar teeth.

In lactation oxytocin acts on the breast ducts causing them to contract when milk is expressed during suckling. The hormone does not have any effect on the secretion of milk by the gland.

Compared with vasopressin an absence of oxytocin has no ill effects. Some replacement may be necessary during labour and lactation only.

2
The Thyroid Gland

Most people are apprehensive about entering hospital, but because each person reacts differently to the situation some appear more nervous than others. One patient may be certain that he will leave hospital in a better state of health, so he has reason to appear confident; others may be less able to hide their anxiety. Some have had previous experience of hospital life which helps them to feel at ease, whereas others feel miserable and strange. Some people are always nervous in new surroundings, and some people appear nervous in any situation, in this last group there will be many who are suffering from some physical or psychological disorder. Occasionally in hospital one meets a new patient whose agitation and distress seems excessive even for the most nervous individual. This patient, frequently a woman, has difficulty in sitting still while the nurse asks the necessary questions on admission. The cup of tea which she is given rattles in the saucer because her hands tremble so badly. She has an intent expression in her eyes and stares earnestly at the nurse whose questions she answers in nervous outbursts of rapid speech. Beads of sweat stand out on her face as though she were facing a terrible ordeal. Her hair is fine and silky and her body and face are thin. This lady is suffering from thyrotoxicosis, a disorder of the thyroid gland.

The thyroid gland lies in the lower part of the neck, just below the cricoid cartilage. It is composed of two oval shaped lobes lying on either side of the trachea which are joined at the front by a narrow part of the gland called the isthmus. In some people the gland has a small additional projection called the pyramidal lobe.

Like all endocrine glands the thyroid gland is an extremely vascular organ. A massive blood supply is essential to allow the secretion to pass into the circulation as quickly as possible when the body requires it. The arterial blood supply comes from the carotid arteries and the subclavian artery, branches of which form the superior and inferior thyroid arteries. The venous return arises from the network of capillaries to form the superior, middle and inferior thyroid veins which flow back into the

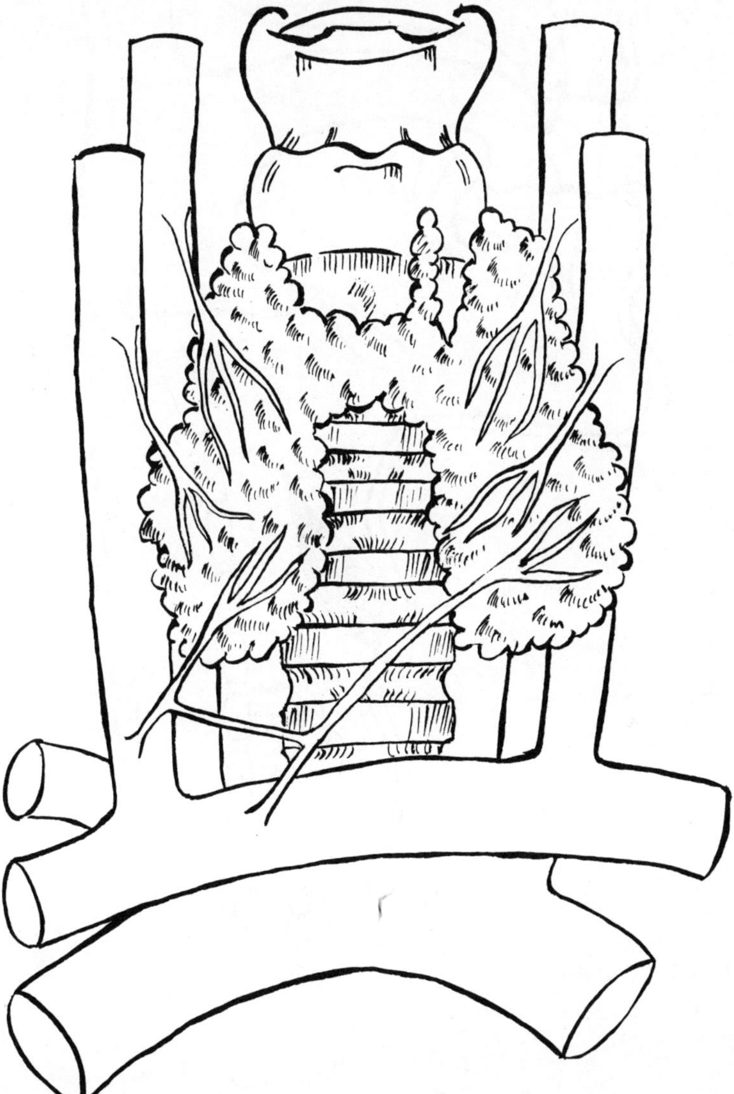

Fig 2:1 Anatomy of the thyroid gland

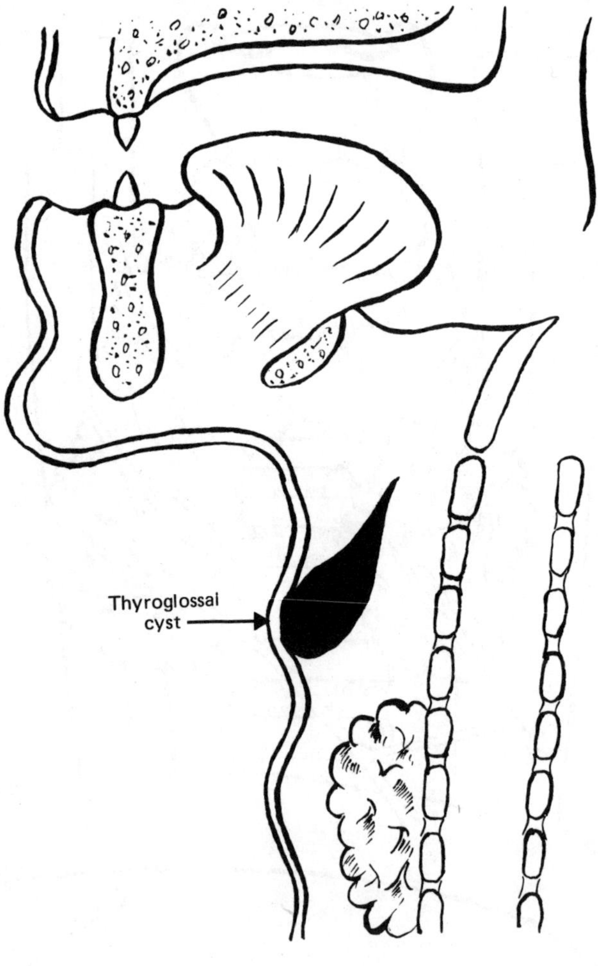

Fig 2:2 Thyroglossal cyst

internal jugular vein. This vascular network is matched by a rich lymphatic supply.

The thyroid gland develops from the floor of the pharynx during the early weeks of foetal life when pouches of tissue grow and descend to fuse and form the gland. The gland originates from a site at the root of the tongue, called the foramen caecum and rudimentary thyroid tissue may be seen in the line of descent, which accounts for the pyramidal lobe. If the descent of thyroid tissue is incomplete fragments of the gland are found at points between the foramen caecum and the site of the normal gland. Such vestiges of tissue may cause noticeable bulges in the neck above the level of the gland and are called thyroglossal cysts, they do not indicate dysfunction. A sinus, and therefore a site for infection, can develop between the undescended portion and the throat. In this situation surgical correction is needed to prevent recurrence of the infection. The special nursing for this procedure is considered with care of the patient having thyroid surgery (page 39).

The gland produces a hormone called thyroxine which acts directly on body tissue by influencing the rate at which cells use energy. Because of the connection between energy and heat it plays a part in body temperature. The activity of the gland is regulated by the trophic hormone, 'thyroid stimulating hormone' (TSH), secreted by the anterior pituitary gland; it is also called thyrotrophin. When the level of thyroxine in the blood is low more TSH is produced stimulating the thyroid gland to increase its secretion of thyroxine. Conversely, excess thyroxine in the blood reduces the supply of TSH which in turn limits the amount of thyroxine produced.

A second hormone, tri-iodothyronine, has been isolated from the thyroid gland. Like thyroxine it speeds up cell function, but its action is quicker and of shorter duration. A third hormone calcitonin, is thought to be secreted by the gland and this has an effect on calcium metabolism.

One active component of thyroxine is iodine. Although this element is to be found in minute fractions in a number of tissues, most of the body's iodine is concentrated in the follicles of the thyroid gland. These are tiny vessels just visible to the naked eye and bound together by connective tissue which contains a jelly-like substance called colloid. It is this colloid which houses the iodine. The amount of colloid varies

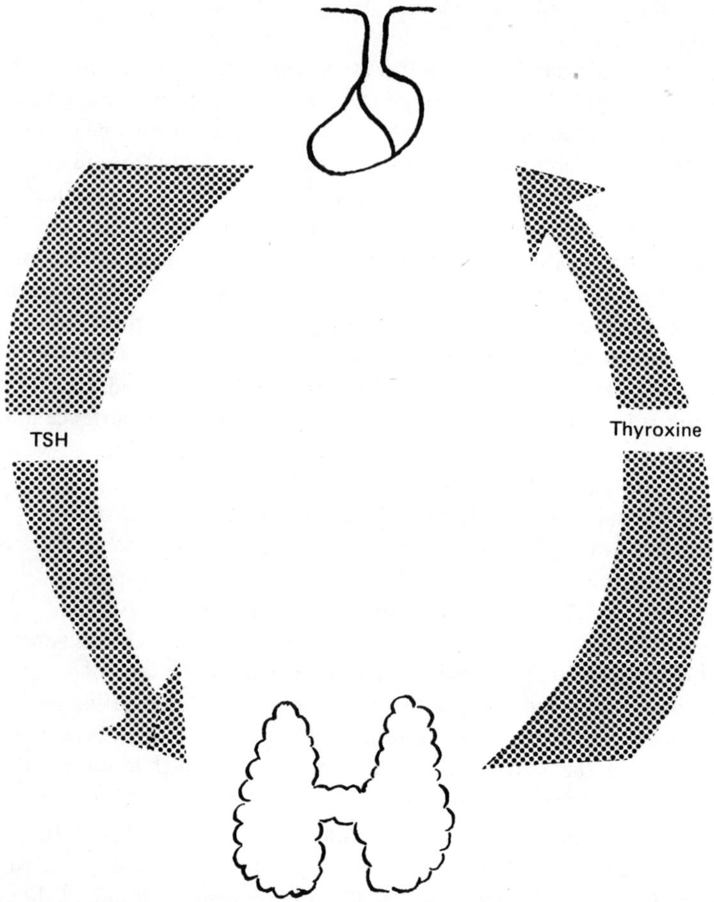

Fig 2:3 Pituitary control

according to the activity of the gland, which may be the reason for glandular enlargement in certain disorders. At this stage the iodine is in loose combination with a protein and is known as thyroglobulin. With the assistance of enzymes this changes to thyroxine.

The body obtains iodine from food particularly milk, sea fish and vegetables grown in soil containing iodine. Rainwater contains no iodine. During the process of digestion iodine passes rapidly from the alimentary tract through the circulation to the thyroid gland. The rate at which iodine is taken up by the gland depends on its activity. This is an important factor in a number of tests for estimating thyroid function.

Goitre

A goitre, which simply means an enlargement of the thyroid gland, can vary from an almost unnoticeable swelling to a degree of enlargement which can cause embarrassment for the patient, both cosmetically and in relation to other structures in the neck. It has a number of causes but is not necessarily an indication of a malfunctioning gland.

Simple goitre

Simple goitre, also called colloid or non-toxic goitre, is attributed to iodine deficiency. Because of the lack of iodine the gland becomes over active in an effort to cope with the demands made upon it. Increased fluid and vascular changes are responsible for the enlargement.

Stress and endocrine changes

This goitre is associated with puberty and adolescent growth. The gland may be only slightly enlarged and is related to changes that occur at this phase of life. The condition is more common in girls in whom such changes are more pronounced. The same enlargement can be seen in pregnant women where considerable endocrine changes are taking place. The subject's thyroid function is normal, and when the stressful cause has passed the enlargement usually disappears spontaneously. Treatment is not needed except in rare cases when the gland does not regress and surgical intervention may be necessary.

Interference in the iodine collecting mechanism
Although iodine is normally taken up by the thyroid gland there are some substances that interfere in the gland's mechanism of iodine collection and inhibit the synthesis of thyroxine. Antithyroid drugs can have this effect, as can certain foods such as cabbage and lettuce when eaten exclusively and in large quantities. They are known as goitrogens. The wide variety of foods eaten today make this a condition that is rarely seen. Should it occur adjustment of the diet under medical supervision should correct it.

Lack of iodine in the diet
People living in certain remote inland areas may develop a goitre and thyroid insufficiency. A number of cases in the past occurred in parts of Derbyshire and Switzerland where supplies of sea fish are limited, there is a consistent lack of iodine in the soil and the water supply is entirely from rainfall. The sea is rich in iodine which is taken up by the fish and also permeates inland into the soil. In areas geographically distant from the sea this natural iodine is absent. When it was discovered that such goitres were the result of iodine lack it was added to prepared table salt, this being a normal constituent of every diet. Once a satisfactory intake is established the activity of the gland is reduced and the goitre diminishes.

Inherited familial defect
To enable iodine to be converted into thyroglobulin – and then thyroxine – certain enzymes are necessary. They are normally present in the body but can be absent through an inherited defect. Medical treatment and correction is required according to the enzymes lacking.

Hyperthyroidism

Oversecretion of thyroxine causing an abnormally high level in the blood is known as hyperthyroidism. It is also called thyrotoxicosis, exophthalmic goitre and Graves' disease. It is frequently associated with enlargement of the gland. The disorder is about eight times more common in women than in men and usually occurs between the ages of puberty and the menopause. The increase in hormone levels is slow and consequently the disease does not manifest itself quickly but develops insidiously over months or years. Thyroxine levels are very closely related to metabolism and any variation will produce widespread changes in body processes; oversecretion of the gland will cause increased activity in all systems of the body. To understand the far reaching effects of hyperthyroidism one must think of all the physiological activities as one interacting process. The heart pumps blood, the lungs exchange gases, the alimentary tract digests, the nervous system controls movement and sensation and each cell carries out an intricate process of living which produces heat and energy. When one of the controlling factors of the system is defective the whole being is changed.

When a thyrotoxic patient is admitted to hospital each of her signs and symptoms can be associated with a disturbance of body function. The first sign the nurse will notice is her extreme anxiety and nervousness, she is unable to sit still for more than a few minutes and her concentration wanders continually. She probably has shaky hands and if her condition is particularly severe she may have a tremor of the head and tongue. She speaks quickly and in spasmodic bursts, she is flushed and obviously sweating profusely. It will be clear that the nurse's most important task is to relieve as much of the anxiety as she can.

Although the patient's symptoms are due to her condition the anxiety is more pronounced in a strange and bustling environment such as a hospital. A nurse can help the patient by being reassuringly calm herself, which is not always easy with an infectiously agitated patient such as this. A quiet, unhurried manner will give the patient the feeling that she is in capable hands. She has probably been worried and upset about her health and her progressively bad 'nerves' over the past months and the presence of someone who understands can be a relief.

If the nurse asks a few questions without appearing to cross examine the patient she will soon discover more about her problems, and avoid the patient having to start the conversation. One of her main worries may be her recent loss of weight. Thyrotoxic patients are invariably thin despite their good appetites and this is often the reason why the patient first consults her doctor. She cannot understand why she has grown so thin when she has been eating well. To the nurse it is obvious that the patient is thinner than she should be as her face looks drawn and haggard, and her neck wrinkled. She appears to be an anxious, exhausted soul, unable to cope any longer.

The patient may insist she is very energetic and yet she finds the tasks she embarks on tiring after a short time. Mentally she is full of energy but somehow her body cannot keep up. Because of her overactive thyroid gland her mental and physical processes are speeded up, which means that although mentally she is prepared to perform a large amount of work, she is too tired physically to manage more than a minimum. To the patient this is alarming, particularly if she has a family to care for and a busy life to organise. When this apprehension is associated with an overactive mind one can appreciate why the characteristic appearance of the hyperthyroid patient is one of continuous anxiety and worry.

The patient's troubles are not confined to this severe state of anxiety. Other systems are disturbed by thyroid dysfunction. Because of overactivity in the alimentary tract she may suffer with diarrhoea. In women the menstrual cycle may be upset causing scanty, irregular periods or complete amenorrhoea. This can be particularly worrying in a young woman to whom any disturbance of her reproductive system can provoke a serious degree of mental trauma.

One of the important problems associated with thyrotoxicosis is the effect on the cardiovascular system, particularly the heart, because the increase in cellular and tissue function causes greater demands on the body's oxygen supply. The lungs can accommodate by raising the respiratory rate – rapid breathing is a common sign in these patients – but the main burden falls on the heart. In the overactive thyroid patient the circulation of oxygen to the tissues needs to be increased. Although this demand may have grown insidiously over many years the heart eventually begins to labour due to the extra pressure placed on it. The patient may complain of palpitations, the apex beat may be forcible and the pulse rapid. This will fluctuate at about 100 to 160 beats per minute and as it is one of the cardinal symptoms it is most important that the nurse records the pulse accurately at regular intervals. Because of the constant overactivity the pulse of the patient does not slow down during sleep, so a sleeping pulse can be a useful record. If the condition was left untreated the strain would continue until the heart failed. This can

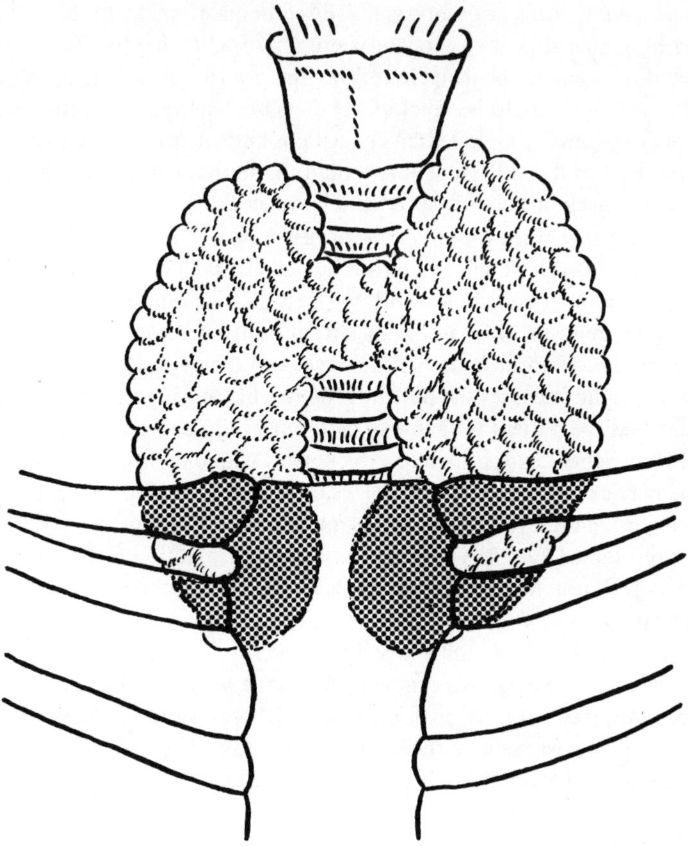

Fig 2:4 Retrosternal goitre

happen in the older patient, or in those whose hearts are damaged from another cause.

There are two further signs associated with hyperthyroidism which the patient may demonstrate to a greater or lesser extent. The first is a goitre which may vary in size. It may be small and barely noticeable or it can reach such large proportions that it creates pressure on the trachea, vocal cords or oesophagus. The consequent difficulty in breathing, speaking or swallowing is not only frightening for the patient but can also be dangerous. The first priority of treatment in this acute situation should be relief of the pressure. One type of goitre where these symptoms become extremely acute is known as a retrosternal goitre. Part of the enlargement is behind the sternum and all the pressure is exerted back on the soft structures in the neck.

The other sign is exophthalmos, or protrusion of the eyeball. Although almost exclusively found in thyrotoxic patients the condition appears to have no direct connection with the dysfunctional thyroid gland. It is caused by deposits of fat in the socket, or orbit, of the eye pushing it forward. It can occur in one or both eyes and the degree of protrusion varies. If mild it causes the patient little trouble but if pushed forward so far that the patient is unable to close the eyelid completely it is called malignant exophthalmos. The patient with exophthalmos of this type may also complain of double vision (diplopia) and loss of eye movement through tension on the rectus muscles. The major problem is that an unprotected eye risks serious injury through infection and corneal scarring. During the day the patient is unable to blink to protect and lubricate her eye but at night she cannot shut it completely and is liable to rub it on the pillow and abrase the cornea.

Although the diagnosis can be made on the patient's physical signs and symptoms it is usual to confirm it by laboratory tests. These have two purposes, to evaluate the activity of the thyroid gland and measure the degree of overactivity, and to estimate cell and tissue function.

Laboratory tests

The activity of the thyroid gland can be measured by the speed with which it collects iodine, and tests have been devised to assess the uptake of traceable iodine. Radioactive iodine is used because it emits gamma rays which can be measured over the body's surface. Radioactive elements are called isotopes, the iodine isotope I^{131} is the substance commonly used in these tests. An isotope's efficiency is measured by its half life, that is the time taken for the activity to be reduced by one half. The half life of I^{131} is seven to eight days, which means that it is extremely effective during the period when estimation of its movements are made. It loses its potency quickly so there is little irradiation risk to the patient. The length of its active life ensures that it is stable when given thus eliminating a possible cause of error in assessing the patient's reaction; it is also inexpensive and easy to use. The alternative isotope is I^{132} which has a half life of only two or three hours. This means the tests must be performed quickly after it is prepared which may not be convenient. It is usually reserved for children and pregnant women in whom radiation doses may be critical.

Many hospital patients feel happier if they know what is involved in any procedure they are subjected to and are able to take an intelligent interest in their treatment. The worrying patient may be alarmed at the thought of a test involving radioactive substances, and therefore the physician may decide the patient should not be told exactly what the material is that will be used in the test. It is most important that the ward staff know of the physician's decision and follow his instructions with care. Nothing is more destructive to good nurse-patient relationships than for the patient to discover something which she feels is vitally important and has not been told. A full but simple explanation can be given to the patient. She can be told that an instrument somewhat like a camera will be used to scan her thyroid gland so that its activity can be measured. If the patient is prepared for these occasions she will be more relaxed and likely to cooperate willingly in the tests and later in the treatment which will then have a greater chance of success.

The test does not require preparation by the patient and it is often performed on patients attending clinics without admission. No pre-testing diet restrictions are necessary, although it is better if the patient has not taken a large meal before the procedure as they may experience some discomfort due to the anxiety. Nor is it necessary for the patient to rest during the hours before the test begins. She is taken to the X-ray department and is given a measured amount of isotope to drink, 10 micrograms is an average adult dose. She is then returned to the ward and continues her daily routine; again no diet or movement restriction is necessary. The patient returns to the X-ray department four hours later for readings to be taken over her thyroid gland using a geiger counter. During this time the iodine has been absorbed through the alimentary system and is being taken up by the thyroid gland. The degree of uptake varies according to the activity of the gland, thus indicating hyperactivity in the thyrotoxic patient. She is returned to the ward and nothing further need be done until the following day, twenty-four hours after the initial dose was given, when a further reading is taken in the X-ray department to assess again the degree of iodine uptake. After the third reading the test is complete.

The patient will consider the test is simple and it does not require her to suffer any painful injection, restrict herself from eating or drinking or take part in any elaborate techniques. This is important as her emotional state should not be taxed more than necessary. Thus a clear picture of what is taking place is all that is needed to get the patient's cooperation.

Because of the radioactive substances used in this test are not strong and have a limited life no specific safeguards are needed to dispose of the patient's excretions. She swallows only a small amount, enough to take diagnostic readings but too little to cause her any harm. However radioactivity can be measured in the urine and the physician may ask for all urine to be collected for checking. It is good practice to instruct the patient in saving her own urine. Patients undergoing investigation in hospital often feel helpless and bored and are pleased to do something useful which gives them a sense of responsibility and participation in their treatment.

The radioactive iodine test estimates the physiological changes in the thyroid gland whilst other tests have been designed to assess changes at cellular and tissue level. The amount of energy expended in the body governs the amount of heat produced. As heat depends on oxygen, the greater the amount of heat the more oxygen is required. Therefore measurement of the body's oxygen intake will correlate fairly accurately with its energy output. Because the use of oxygen varies with activity a test to measure the oxygen used is only valid when compared with fixed standard of movement. It has been found the most reliable measurement is made when the body is at rest.

A test has been designed to estimate the number of Calories used in necessary body processes, eg heart beating, respiration and peristalsis. Because it is the lowest number of Calories the body requires for metabolism when the subject is at rest it is called basal metabolic rate (BMR). Specific standards of BMR have been calculated according to age, weight, sex and area of body surface. The result of the test is compared with the appropriate standard which indicates whether the patient is above the normal level. Unfortunately the ideal situation is rarely achieved as the slightest movement can cause deviations which give an inaccurate reading and make the assessment difficult. The BMR test on its own is considered too unstable for positive diagnosis and may be used in conjunction with the radioactive iodine test.

It cannot be emphasised too strongly how important it is to be rested and relaxed for this test, which is difficult with a thyrotoxic patient. An explanation of the procedure and the reason for doing it will help to allay the patient's fears. In this test the patient has a nose and mouth clip over her face which can be frightening if unexpected. A trial with a nurse in which the patient handles and fits the nose clip and mouthpiece herself can give useful foreknowledge which will help her to relax during the actual test.

The patient's physical preparation begins the night before the test. If sedation is prescribed it may be given earlier than usual as nothing is taken by mouth after 10 pm and the patient requires a good night's sleep. The following morning she should be disturbed as little as possible and should not get out of bed to wash or visit the toilet. Some patients object to bedpans and the nurse should use her discretion in deciding whether it would be easier and less disturbing for the patient to use the toilet in a wheelchair.

The test measures the amount of oxygen used when at rest. To do this the patient breathes continuously into a tube using the nose clip and mouthpiece to ensure that all gases of respiration pass through the machine, the quantity of gas being measured on a spirometer. Throughout this time the patient should move only when necessary and must not talk. To ensure a peaceful atmosphere the test is best conducted in a quiet room with the minimum number of people present. When the test is complete the patient may return to her bed and is given a meal.

Only a small percentage of circulating thyroid hormone is free to act on cells and tissues, the remainder is bound to plasma proteins. The free hormone is a small fraction and cannot be measured but the larger protein bound part can be measured by laboratory analysis. This is the protein bound iodine test and requires a blood sample from the patient.

Treatment

When the tests are complete and the diagnosis is confirmed the physician can decide which form of treatment is to be given. The patient may be feeling more anxiety than before knowing that her recovery depends on the treatment. She will be aware that her problem is deeper than she had thought and she will realise that it is necessary to remain in hospital for proper care and observation during the initial stages to ensure that the cure is permanent.

Treatment of hyperthyroidism aims to stabilise the patient's body processes and restore normal metabolism. The primary concern is to reduce the strain on the patient's heart, which can be damaged irreparabl if the condition is neglected. Three types of treatment are available.

1 Antithyroid drugs
2 Radioactive iodine
3 Surgery

Antithyroid drugs

Drugs in the antithyroid group act by blocking the production of thyroxine from the gland, causing a reduction in metabolism. Physical changes with this treatment are slow and there are a number of observations necessary before drug therapy begins to aid in the assessment of progress. The doctor may order a laboratory analysis of the patient's blood, a picture of the normal blood fractions is needed to compare with specimens during treatment to ensure that continuous drug absorption does not produce damaging changes. Both before and during treatment nursing observations will include regular, accurate recordings of the patient's pulse, respiratory rate, blood pressure and weight. Measurement of the patient's neck circumference will be made in the initial stages of investigation, and this will be repeated when treatment begins for comparative estimation of the goitre size.

Drugs of the thiocarbamide group are most commonly used for

treating hyperthyroidism; of these Carbimazole is considered most reliable. Treatment begins with 10 mg three times daily by mouth. The patient will notice no change in her condition for two or three weeks, after which she becomes more relaxed and cooperative. Her physical disturbances will gradually decline and she will slowly gain weight. Once the maximum improvement has been reached the dosage may be reduced. The body's responses to treatment is slow and weekly improvement will vary according to the degree of hyperthyroidism.

Side effects of drug therapy are rare, however when they occur serious problems can result. One complication is agranulocytosis, a blood disorder in which there is a reduction in the white cells. Sore throat and joint pains are early indicators of this condition and the patient is advised to report to her doctor when any of these signs appear, however mild they may seem. If the complication is proved positive the antithyroid drug should be stopped and alternative treatment given as permanent damage can result. Antithyroid drugs can also cause an increase in the size of a goitre which could present pressure symptoms if the goitre is retrosternal.

Medical nursing care

Certain aspects of care are particularly important in the medical treatment of thyrotoxicosis. The first is rest, both physical and mental. Considering the changes created in this condition and the stress suffered by the patient rest is a difficult thing to achieve, but it is essential if the strain on the heart is to be reduced. It is easier to induce an atmosphere of calm and tranquillity if the patient is nursed in a small, less busy ward than one devoted to the acutely ill where nurses scurry about in a pre-occupied manner. An agitated thyroid patient can also be a disturbing influence to other patients, so on both counts a small ward is the best solution.

The nurse should plan her work so that all necessary tasks are performed on the patient at one time, instead of subjecting her to a routine of care at odd times. This relates to the physical problems which the nurse should bear in mind when caring for the patient. Because she is overactive her senses will tend to be overacute. Her skin is more sensitive to touch which calls for greater skill in bed bathing or giving care that involves handling or touching the skin. Bright lights are blinding, sudden noise is nerve shattering, and the nurse should do all in her power to protect her patient from such miseries.

A thyrotoxic patient will constantly complain of the heat, she will want to sleep with few bedclothes and the window wide open. It is the nurse's duty to make sure this need for fresh air is kept to moderate levels and that the patient is not exposed to draughts. Although she is producing a greater amount of heat she is still subject to the same chills as others. She may sleep with her arms outside of the bedclothes, this is useful if the nurse is stealthy in taking the radial pulse when she is asleep. Because of her sensitivity it may be difficult to do this without waking her and it is often easier to take the pulse by watching the temporal artery which should show clearly as the patient tends to be thin and blood vessels are more pronounced.

If the patient's heart is affected drugs may be needed. Atrial fibrillation is commonly encountered and for this digoxin will be prescribed to produce a stronger, slower beat. Pulse recordings are important with patients taking this drug as an unduly slowed pulse will indicate overdosage. If her heart is failing the patient may have oedema, due to a poor venous return so diuretics will be given to remove excess fluid.

Exophthalmos can cause problems if the protrusion is so bad that scarring of the eye is liable to occur. The patient may be troubled by what they describe as itching over the surface of the eye, and Soframycin 0.5 per cent or Guanethidine five per cent, eye drops can relieve this successfully. Hypersensitivity to light can be disturbing for a patient with severe exophthalmos and relief can be given if shields are fitted to the sides of her spectacles to cut out extra rays of light.

The diet of a thyrotoxic patient requires careful control. When first admitted she will have an enormous appetite and as she is so energetic she needs the extra Calories. The diet should be nourishing and rich in dairy products such as milk and eggs. If her digestion is affected the diet should contain less rich, indigestible food to reduce discomfort. Because she will perspire heavily the nurse should keep careful observation on her fluid intake, there should always be a drink on the patient's locker and an intake and output chart may be necessary. Her appetite and need for fluids will diminish as treatment progresses and the nurse should make adjustment as recovery takes place.

Radioactive iodine

Where drugs have proved ineffective or unsuitable other forms of treatment are considered. One of these is radioactive iodine which has a very limited but effective use. This treatment uses the thyroid gland's ability to trap iodine. I^{131} is given to the patient in larger doses than is used for diagnostic tests. The iodine is taken up by the gland and the radiation emitted causes permanent damage to the gland tissues, resulting in a diminished thyroxine output. This degree of radiation is not generally harmful to the body but can have serious effects on the reproductive system. Because of this it cannot be used in children or patients during the reproductive age and is reserved for some patients in the older age groups.

Surgery

Certain cases of hyperthyroidism are best treated surgically. These include those who fail to respond to medical treatment, patients who have a massive goitre causing pressure symptoms and those cases considered unsuitable for drug or radioactive iodine therapy. The gland may be partly removed (partial thyroidectomy) or completely removed (total thyroidectomy). Whenever possible partial thyroidectomy is performed because of the complications caused by a total loss of all thyroid secretions.

Once it is decided that surgery is the treatment of choice the patient is admitted for special pre-operative preparation to reduce the chance of complications to a minimum. When the gland is overactive and enlarged it is highly vascular and tense. In order to make it smaller and more friable – and therefore easier to manage at operation – the patient is given a course of antithyroid drugs, such as Carbimazole. Although the effect of the drug is to reduce the gland in size it becomes more vascular than before. To counteract this the drug is stopped about one week before operation and replaced by a course of iodine with potassium iodide (Lugol's iodine). This reduces the vascularity sufficiently to minimise the risk of haemorrhage at operation.

The operation presents problems because of the danger to adjacent structures such as the parathyroid glands and the laryngeal nerves. It is also difficult to assess the amount of thyroid tissue to be removed to allow normal body function without risk of hypothyroidism or hyperthyroidism in the future.

The patient may be admitted into a surgical ward or transferred from a medical ward following investigation and diagnosis. The patient will present a similar picture to that described earlier in the chapter (page 29) with the added worry of impending surgery causing her anxiety to be more acute. Her vivid imaginings may be made worse by lurid tales of operations that she may have heard or read. Because of the extreme stress and apprehension of a patient undergoing this surgery they may be asked to come into hospital earlier than other surgical patients to allow time to become accustomed to the ward and its routine. Apart from the pre-operative drug preparation the patient is given the opportunity to know the ward staff which may allay her anxiety.

The surgeon will discuss the operation with the patient and explain it to her. It is important than an adequate explanation is made as it is necessary for the patient to sign an operation consent form before surgery is carried out. If the surgeon does not ask the patient to sign the consent form it is the responsibility of the nursing staff to ensure that the form is completed, and witnessed by the person who is present when the patient signs her name. An important point of this procedure is that the form must be signed before the patient is given her premedication for theatre. She must be completely aware of the contents and implications of the form she is signing.

Pre-operative preparation will include sedatives to reduce the patient's tension and allow her rest, cardiac drugs if the heart is affected, chest X-ray and examination of the vocal cords. On the day of operation she will have her axillae and upper arms shaved (and chest if the patient is a male). Followed by a bath, gowning and general pre-operative measures. The patient's fears will be at their greatest about the time of premedication, which will have a relaxing effect. The ward nurse should accompany her to theatre and stay with her until she is anaesthetised.

Post operative care. It is common practice today for all patients to return from theatre following recovery of consciousness in the recovery room. However, if the patient is still unconscious on returning to the ward she should be nursed flat and on her side until her cough reflex returns, and she must not be left unobserved due to the risk of an obstructed airway. If she vomits the nurse will need to keep the wound area clean and free from debris. On recovery from anaesthetic her head may be supported by one pillow and gradually progress until a sitting position is adopted with the head and neck well supported. It is important at this time that she does not jerk her head or twist her neck.

She may encounter some difficulty in speaking and swallowing for the first few days but the staff can reassure her that this problem will pass as the operation site heals and tension and localised oedema are reduced. She may have sips of water during the immediate post-operative period but it is extremely painful to swallow and frequent mouth care may be needed. Apart from the initial pain it is not difficult for the patient to take fluids by mouth, therefore an intravenous infusion is rarely used.

Normal post-operative observations are commenced and recorded, including temperature, pulse and respiration rate. The pulse is again important and a record should be kept every quarter of an hour at first, then half hourly for the following twelve hours. The nurse should report immediately any irregularity at once as it may indicate heart involvement to which the patient is prone, it could also show possible haemorrhage.

The patient should start to lose her thyrotoxic symptoms now that the greater part of the organ has been removed. It takes some while for all the symptoms to disappear completely. She may still suffer from the heat during the post-operative period and it may be necessary to remove blankets if asked. If the patient is perspiring excessively tepid sponging can be comforting, again avoidance of draughts is important.

It is common practice to close the edges of a thyroidectomy wound with clips or alternate clips and sutures and the dressing is held in place by an Elastoplast strip. Some surgeons prefer to close the wound completely while others insert a small drain which is removed after forty-eight hours. At this time the wound is inspected to ensure that the clips and sutures are satisfactory and the wound edges are not gaping.

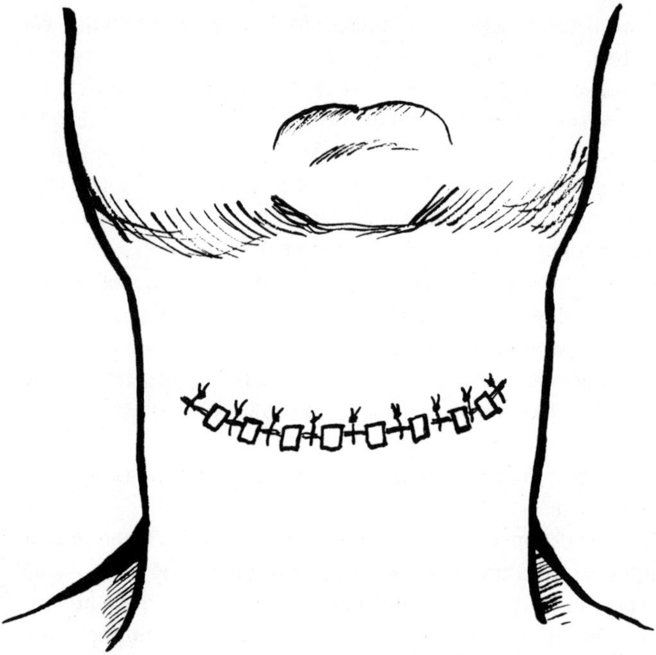

Fig 2:5 Thyroidectomy wound

Alternate clips or sutures are removed on the third post-operative day, and the remainder on the fifth or sixth day if the wound is clean and healing well.

If no complications appear during the immediate post-operative period the patient may sit out of bed from the second day following operation, and will be discharged about the tenth day if her progress is maintained. There are several complications that can arise following thyroidectomy, the nurse should be aware of these and make observations accordingly.

Haemorrhage. Haemorrhage will not be outwardly obvious because of the patient's dressing, but its effect can be seen at once. The clips and sutures keep the wound closed which prevents the escape of blood, this causes pressure, the patient has difficulty in breathing and swallowing and appears shocked. This is an emergency situation and immediate steps are necessary to relieve pressure on the trachea. The clips and sutures must be removed and clots extracted from the wound. It is preferable that such action is taken by a doctor but the ward nurse should be prepared to carry out this procedure if necessary. Because of the urgency to regain a clear airway it may be necessary for an aseptic technique to be disregarded. Speed is essential and all ward nurses should be aware of the importance of reporting any breathing difficulty in this patient. When the sutures are removed and the patient relieved of the respiratory embarassment she will be returned to theatre for location of the bleeding points and resuturing.

Thyrotoxic crisis. This complication is rare, but when it occurs it may be extremely serious particularly in the patient who has heart complications. Release of excessive amounts of thyroxine is one cause and is likely to take place if the patient has not been adequately prepared with drugs before operation. The patient displays all the signs of acute hyperthyroidism, becomes agitated with a raised temperature and pulse. The signs are highly exaggerated and the patient's change should be reported immediately. A sedative may be prescribed to reduce the activity, digoxin may be ordered as fibrillation can occur and antithyroid drugs are used to control the glandular activity.

Atrial fibrillation. The patient whose heart is affected by thyrotoxicosis may develop atrial fibrillation spontaneously during the postoperative period. It may not be connected with thyroid crisis and can be an isolated symptom. Early detection depends on the nurse's assessment and recording of the pulse. It should be calculated with care, it is not enough to count the number of beats per minute, strength and rhythm are important and should be noted. If the pulse is irregular or the beats produced in an uncontrolled manner the doctor should be informed and action taken.

Continued loss of voice. It is to be expected that the patient will have a sore throat and a hoarse voice for the first few days following operation. Steam inhalations can be given to aid recovery and relieve oedema of the throat. If the hoarseness persists the surgeon will investigate the possibility of damage to the recurrent laryngeal nerve which could be permanent.

Parathyroid involvement. The parathyroid glands are attached to the posterior aspect of the thyroid and although efforts are made to avoid them during operation they may be damaged. If parathyroid secretion is impaired it will take several days for the symptoms to appear, the patient will complain of muscle tightening and the nurse will notice twitching movements, particularly around the mouth. This is a sign that a condition called tetany is developing (see chapter   ) and will need urgent correction.

Other causes of goitre

Simple and thyrotoxic goitre have been discussed, there are several other causes of goitre development.

Acute thyroiditis

Acute inflammation of the thyroid gland is uncommon but can occur with upper respiratory tract infection with staphylococcal or streptococcal organisms particularly if suppuration takes place. Women are more affected than men, the gland becomes swollen and painful to touch and the patient may have dysphagia. The condition can last for several weeks and the patient recovers spontaneously. An anti-inflammatory drug such as prednisone can aid the inflammation to recover quickly.

Chronic thyroiditis (Hashimoto's disease)

This also is a disease affecting females more than males, mainly between the ages of thirty-five to fifty-five years. Although the condition is called thyroiditis there are no infecting organisms as it is an auto-immune disease. Thyroid antibody cells are produced in the patient's body which invade and gradually destroy the gland. This lessens the secretion of thyroxine as the gland becomes non-functional until secretion ceases. In an effort to compensate for the diminished supply of thyroxine the active part of the gland enlarges, producing a goitre. Treatment consists of oral thyroxine as replacement therapy and if the goitre causes pressure symptoms surgery may be needed.

Carcinoma of the thyroid gland
Malignant tumours of the thyroid gland account for only 200–400 deaths each year, women over forty form the largest group although it can affect children and young people. The early symptoms are neck discomfort, voice changes, hoarseness, dysphagia and dyspnoea. Treatment is by total thyroidectomy coupled with radiotherapy. Drug replacement is necessary to avoid acute hypothyroidism.

Hypothyroidism

Hypothyroidism, or myxoedema, like many thyroid disorders is more commonly found in females, particularly those near or past the menopause. It is an undersecretion of thyroxine causing the metabolism to slow down below the normal level of efficiency. It usually has a slow onset over many years unless created by some sudden change to glandular activity such as total thyroidectomy. Clinically it is the thyrotoxic picture reversed, instead of the fast acting nervous person the myxoedematous patient is slow and lethargic.

There are two types of hypothyroidism – primary and secondary. Primary failure is an inefficient gland without loss of the pituitary influence. Secondary failure is due to loss of TSH (thyroid stimulating hormone)

Causes of primary failure include:

Irradiation
Treatment of thyrotoxicosis with radioactive isotopes (see page 39) can result in the gland become incompetent several years later.

Surgery
Following a partial thyroidectomy myxoedema can develop if the remaining thyroid tissue fails to secrete sufficient thyroxine.

Idiopathic hypothyroidism

Most hypothyroid patients have no known cause for their deficiency. It may be associated with acute thyroiditis several years before but this is not the only cause as many patients have no previous history of thyroid disorders.

Auto-immunity

Chronic thyroiditis eventually results in loss of all active thyroid tissue.

Drugs

Certain groups of drugs, including tolbutamide and para-amino salicylic acid may depress the thyroid gland. Although anti-thyroid drugs reduce natural hormone production no permanent loss of function is caused for when the drug is stopped the gland returns to normal.

The patient's slow movements will be the first thing the nurse will notice when she is admitted. Like the thyrotoxic patient her concentration will be minimal, but in this case it is not due to excess activity but complete lack of interest in her surroundings. People may have remarked how slow she is even to do the simplest tasks. They think she is lazy yet to her everything is such a dreadful effort. She now dresses in the warmest, thickest clothes and yet always seems cold. She may be anaemic, her skin is dry and coarse, she is puffy around the eyes and her scanty hair is lustreless and brittle. Her appetite is small yet she is putting on weight steadily and will complain of constipation. When the nurse takes her temperature it will register one to two degree less than normal and her pulse and respiration rates are reduced. This is a typical picture of the myxoedema patient admitted to hospital for confirmation of the diagnosis and to begin treatment.

Laboratory tests

Diagnosis of hypothyroidism is confirmed using the same tests as for thyrotoxicosis – assessment of BMR, iodine uptake and protein bound iodine. In the myxoedematous patient the results will be reversed. The BMR test will show a reduced level of tissue and cellular activity, iodine uptake will show a slower uptake rate, the counter reading being taken over a longer period and protein bound iodine levels will be low.

Treatment

Once the diagnosis is confirmed treatment is started as soon as possible. The aim is to raise the patient's metabolic level to a near normal degree and maintain it permanently. This means that drug therapy will continue for the rest of the patient's life.

Treatment is no longer by the administration of thyroid extract but by taking oral thyroxine daily. This drug is produced synthetically and is completely safe if precautions are observed. In the patient whose body has been functioning abnormally slowly for several years any sudden rise in hormone would produce an equally fast increase in metabolism. Most organs could adapt to this but the effect on the heart could be dangerous and heart failure could follow.

To avoid this, the dose of thyroxine is low at first and is increased gradually. Treatment is started with 0.05mg daily and increased by 0.05mg daily each week until a daily dose of 0.2 to 0.3mg is reached. During this time the patient's improvement and physical condition are regularly assessed. The nurse is required to record temperature, pulse, respiration and blood pressure with accuracy. The patient may develop diarrhoea or tachycardia while the dose is rising and these facts should be reported immediately for adjustment of the drug.

Cretinism

Congenital thyroid deficiency produces a state of retarded mental and physical growth known as cretinism. During the first few weeks of life the lack of hormone will not become apparent as the baby receives thyroxine from the mother's circulation. Signs of cretinism appear from the sixth week of life. The baby fails to develop both physically and mentally and its body functions and activities are abnormally slow.

The baby may be brought to the doctor because of its failure to thrive and to reach the usual milestones. He is slow and retarded with sluggish mental and physical reactions. The normal child's grasping, laughing, crawling and walking phases are conspicuously delayed. His heart and pulse rate are slow, the bridge of his nose appears flat and his tongue is large and protrudes from his mouth. He may appear to have a slight goitre. A distended abdomen, frequently with an umbilical hernia is a common feature, as is constipation and the yellow, cold dry skin so typical of cretinism.

The earlier treatment is commenced the greater is the chance of correcting the child's retardation, and of a normal life in the future. Therefore it is imperative that a treatment regime is begun immediately the diagnosis is made. The thyroxine dose must be built up cautiously as in the adult patient and the child must continue to take the drug for the remainder of his life. The success of the treatment is assessed by the growth and intelligence of the child as he develops. Before the discovery of hormone therapy cretinous children were doomed to a short and miserable life. Today the outlook for them is good, provided that treatment is started in the early months of life.

3
Parathyroid Glands

'At first I just seemed to have weak ankles and I felt very unsteady when going down stairs but gradually this muscle weakness got worse and worse until after a year or so even my walking was affected. I had to use my arms to lift myself up from a chair and it was quite hard work to lift my legs off the ground when I got into bed at night. My elbows were very painful too and for some reason my eyelids began to droop. My doctor noticed a swelling in my neck and arranged for me to have X-rays. Apparently they showed a weakness in the bones. He said they were not opaque as they should be in an X-ray. They were almost transparent so in the skull X-ray the brain could be seen quite clearly. He said I had something called hyperparathyroidism.'

The lady who made this statement was suffering from a disorder of the parathyroid glands. These consist of four small oval bodies embedded in the posterior aspect of the thyroid gland – hence the name, para means by the side of or beyond. They are found in the lateral lobes of the thyroid gland and are positioned in pairs.

Because of the close relationship between the thyroid and parathyroid glands they share a common blood supply from branches of the superior and inferior thyroid arteries. A nerve supply arises from the cervical sympathetic ganglia which does not affect the function of the gland directly but causes its blood vessels to dilate or contract. In foetal life the rudimentary pharynx forms a number of pouches that are destined to grow into specific organs and tissues. They are eventually found in sites through the head, neck and upper thorax and include the tonsils, thymus, thyroid and parathyroid glands. The growth and purpose of each pouch is well defined. The upper parathyroid glands develop from the fourth pouch while the lower glands develop from the third pouch. Because of this origin the parathyroid glands are sometimes referred to by numbers which can lead to confusion for nurses reading a doctor's notes. Thus the upper parathyroid glands become parathyroid IV and the lower parathyroid glands are parathyroid III.

The hormone secreted by the glands is called parathyroid hormone

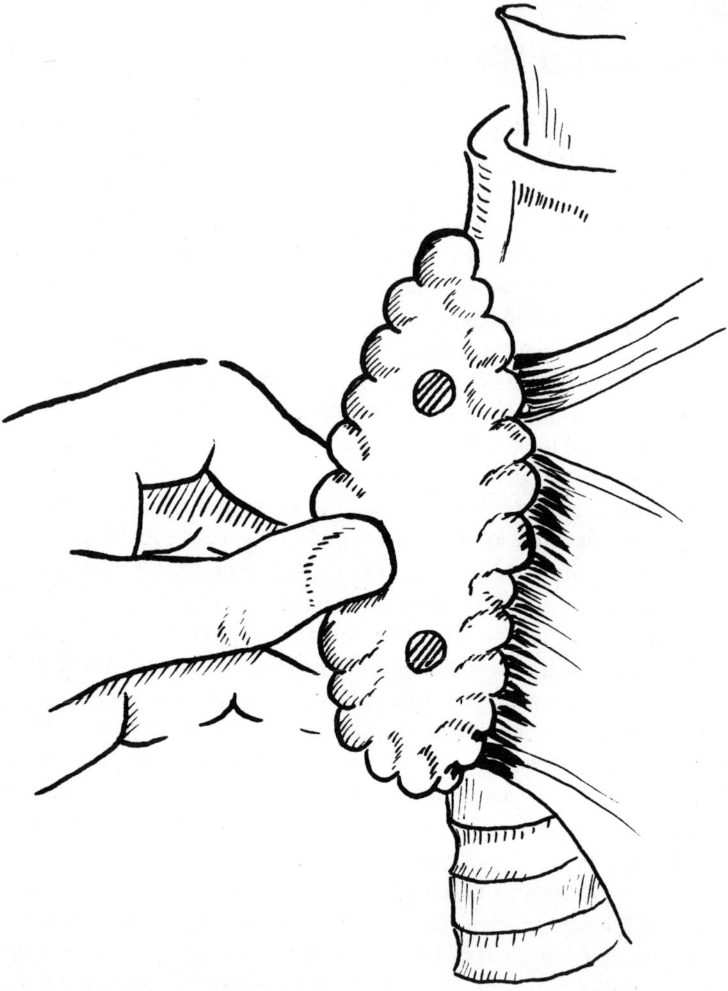

Fig 3:1 The parathyroid glands

(PTH) and, as with the pancreas, its rate of secretion is governed by circulating substances in the blood. In the parathyroid gland the controlling fraction is calcium and the amount of PTH secreted is determined by the level of plasma calcium. If the level falls the gland is stimulated and if it rises the secretion is diminished. The level of phosphorus is in inverse proportion to calcium which means that when the calcium level falls the phosphorus level rises by an equivalent amount. Should the calcium level rise the phosphorus will be reduced by the same proportion. A second hormone affecting the parathyroid glands has been isolated which lowers the serum calcium. Originally called calcitonin, recent studies show it to be secreted by the thyroid gland, because of this it has been renamed thyrocalcitonin (TCH).

The action of PTH is not completely understood, but it is responsible for maintaining the level of blood calcium and the excretion of excess phosphorus through the kidneys. It is assumed that the normal serum calcium level (9–11mg per 100ml of blood) is the result of a balance between a regular dietary intake of calcium and a stable parathyroid gland. Phosphorus levels are controlled by the action of PTH on the distal tubules of the kidney where reabsorption of phosphorus takes place.

In the body calcium plays an important part in the formation of bones and teeth. It is necessary for the passage of nerve impulses, notably at the neuromuscular junctions. If the level of calcium is persistently low the nerve control of muscle is lost. Muscle tissue itself also needs a constant supply of calcium to function efficiently, particularly cardiac muscle with its controlled, regular contractions. Finally calcium is essential for the clotting of blood.

The main sources of calcium are cow's milk, green vegetables and bread, the average daily intake of calcium is 1 to 2gms. It is absorbed through the wall of the alimentary tract and any excess is excreted. Vitamin D is vital for absorption to take place, without it calcium cannot be taken into the body however high the concentration in the food may be.

Phosphorus is an important constituent of all body cells being concerned with the production of energy and normal cell function. Inorganic phosphates in the form of calcium phosphate also form part of the structure of bones. Phosphorus is found in milk and dairy produce.

The two disorders of the parathyroid glands are hyperparathyroidism and hypoparathyroidism.

Hyperparathyroidism

This is a condition in which an excessive amount of PTH is secreted. Some patients oversecrete for no apparent reason although the glands may enlarge, in others the disorder is due to the presence of small tumours. Other conditions such as chronic renal disease, intestinal malabsorption and lack of vitamin D in the diet can raise the level of PTH as they may lead to constantly low levels of plasma calcium and this overstimulates the glands.

The oversecretion of hormone causes calcium and phosphorus to be mobilised from the bones and lost through the kidneys in large amounts. Because of these changes the patient will present signs and symptoms related to the functions of calcium in the body.

The patient will be admitted to a medical ward for investigation and initial treatment. She may appear drowsy and lethargic with a distinct weakness of the limbs. The nurse admitting her should see that the new patient has a comfortable and safe place to sit, her bones may be very fragile and could be broken easily by accidental falls.

It is usual for the patient to drink a great deal and pass large amounts of urine during the early stages of treatment. This is necessary for the kidneys to filter and excrete the extra amount of mineral salts being lost. She may feel nauseated and reluctant to drink, a sign associated with high calcium levels, in this instance the nurse should encourage the patient to drink as much as possible. If nausea continues the nurse can save the patient a great deal of embarrassment by ensuring that there is a bowl within easy reach in case she should vomit. The patient's appetite is an important observation of the nurse. Her frequent nausea may prevent her from eating correctly but a well balanced diet is essential. Encouragement is needed and she should be given small, attractive meals of easily digested food in preference to large portions which she cannot manage. A further reason for the patient to take regular meals is a complication of hyperparathyroidism, a peptic ulcer which can be irritated by long periods without food.

If the patient had polyuria before coming into hospital, observations will be necessary to detect dehydration including loss of elasticity of the skin, sunken eyes and a dirty mouth. An ample fluid intake is needed and regular mouth care in the less able patient. The patient may complain of dizziness, particularly when bending. Loss of calcium from the bones means they are brittle and easily broken thus vertigo is an added risk to an already accident prone patient. The nurse should ensure that someone is with her when she walks in the ward and she should be warned not to bend down for any reason. If she drops something on the floor she should not hesitate to ask to have it picked up for her. This is very important in the elderly who may be frail when in good health and are at particular risk. Because of the effect on nervous tissue the hyperparathyroid patient may show signs of mental disturbance, mild agitation, confusion or depression. In this instance careful watch is needed as she is more likely to fall in such a disturbed phase.

Patients with hyperparathyroidism admitted for treatment may be given tests to confirm the diagnosis. These include estimation of blood serum calcium, X-ray examination of the bones and renal tract and bone biopsy to estimate calcium loss.

Laboratory testing of plasma calcium is a useful diagnostic aid once the dietary intake of calcium has been established. It is best achieved after a period of fasting, because absorption following a meal can affect the readings. The nurse should give the patient a simple explanation for the test and the reason for fasting. When she realises that it is necessary and helpful to her treatment she will cooperate more willingly. It causes the patient little hardship to fast overnight and have the test early in the morning followed by a late breakfast.

X-ray examination will show the density of bone tissue and whether calcium has been mobilised and withdrawn, leaving the bones thin or mis-shapen. Straight X-ray or intravenous pyelography pictures may also demonstrate calcium deposits or calculi that form in the kidneys. If hyperparathyroidism is confirmed at this stage there will be no need for a bone biopsy which could cause the patient unnecessary stress.

If the increased secretion of PTH is caused by an adenoma the affected gland can be removed surgically. Following this operation the nurse should watch carefully for signs of the reverse condition – hypoparathyroidism. This can take place if too much parathyroid tissue is removed. It is difficult for the surgeon to estimate precisely how much of the gland is causing the primary condition.

In chronic renal disease the normal passage of calcium through the kidney and its reabsorption in the tubules is inefficient so that much of the calcium may be lost in the urine. It is also thought that in certain chronic renal disorders there is some resistance to the absorption of vitamin D which is a necessary factor in the utilisation of calcium in the diet. Treatment in these cases is directed towards curing or stabilising the renal disorder, which is often difficult or impossible. In an effort to correct the parathyroid disturbance supplements of calcium and vitamin D may be given in addition to the normal diet. Hyperparathyroidism associated with intestinal malabsorption presents a similar clinical picture. Vitamin D is a fat soluble vitamin therefore any disease in which fat absorption is impaired will influence the absorption of the D vitamin. Treatment is difficult as the cause of malabsorption is not easily identified.

One other classically important reason for hyperparathyroidism is lack of vitamin D in the diet causing the disease rickets. This is a condition showing malformation of the bones, particularly the long, weight bearing bones. Rickets is rarely seen in developed countries today because of the care given to growing children and the general improvement in diet and housing. Social and medical history shows that it was not rare in the poor communities of Britain during the nineteenth century. Ordinary food contains sufficient vitamin D for normal requirements and this can be supplemented by a natural supply through exposure of the skin to sunlight. Although occasional cases of rickets are still seen at hospital outpatient clinics they are from physiological causes and are not dietary in origin. Treatment is often by exposure to sunlight, particularly the ultra violet rays, which are essential for the production of vitamin D in conjunction with a substance found under the skin called ergosterol.

Hypoparathyroidism

Undersecretion of the parathyroid glands can be caused by idopathic atrophy, by damage from failure of the blood supply, or through surgical interference.

A typical patient with hypoparathyroidism is a woman who has had a partial thyroidectomy some time before. When seen by the nurse on re-admission her thyroidectomy scar may still be obvious – really acute cases will develop during the post operative period. She will complain of painful muscles and uncontrolled spasms which affect the hands and feet (carpo-pedal spasms). She will have tingling of the fingers, toes and small muscles around the mouth. This patient will require careful observation during the critical period before treatment becomes effective. Because of the defective muscular control she is liable to fall easily and may be subject to epileptiform convulsions. These falling attacks come on without warning and she should be accompanied when walking in the ward or going to the bathroom. At other times she can be settled comfortably in a suitable chair to reduce the risk of accident. It is important to point out to the patient that her safety is the nurse's priority and that she will not object to being called from other tasks. The patient must not be reticent in asking for help in this situation.

Tetany

This condition of increased neuromuscular excitability causing twitchings, carpo-pedal spasms and convulsions is called tetany. It only becomes apparent if the blood calcium is at an extremely low level. If the amount of calcium is at a less reduced level mild hypoparathyroidism will result. Because the imbalance is not acute the patient will suffer from different symptoms. On admission she may appear depressed and not very communicative. Physically the nurse will notice how easily she gets tired, she needs a rest after the least exertion – a walk through the ward or a visit to the X-ray department. Any movements made during the course of her admission will be slow and more laborious. Occasionally she may complain of cramp in the lower limbs which massage and movement does not help.

Tests for this disorder are similar to those used in the diagnosis of hyperparathyroidism. A reduced level of PTH causes a low plasma calcium which is indicated by blood tests. Because calcium is related to the efficiency of muscle tissue an electrocardiograph will demonstrate variations of cardiac muscle function. X-ray of bones will indicate changes in skeletal structure.

Nurses may notice the physician perform two particular tests on the patient during the physical examination.

1 Chvostek's sign

When the facial nerve is tapped just above the angle of the jaw a positive response would be severe twitching of the facial muscles on that side, in particular at the corners of the mouth.

2 Trousseau's sign

When a sphygmomanometer is applied to the patient's arm in the usual manner and inflated above the systolic pressure on acute muscular spasm will cause the patient to flex the wrist whilst the fingers are flexed at the metacarpophalangeal joints and extended at the interphalangeal joints.

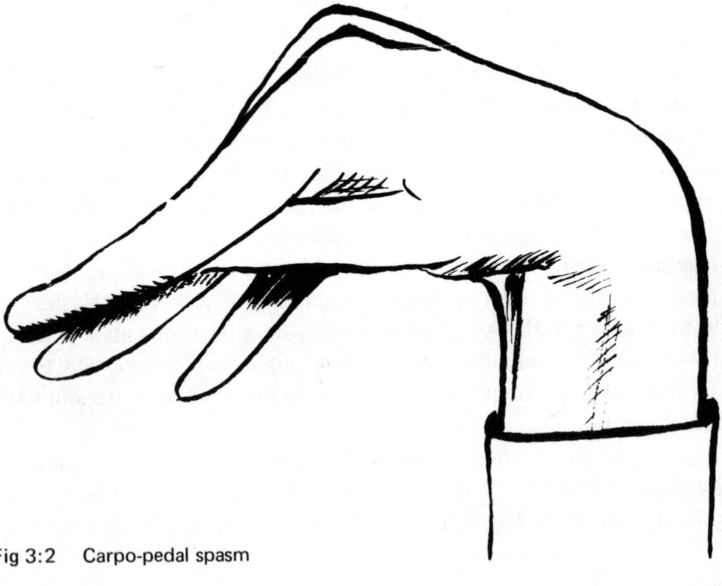

Fig 3:2 Carpo-pedal spasm

Most of the physical symptoms of the hypoparathyroid patient can be associated with the inefficiency of muscle tissue. A normal level of plasma calcium is necessary for controlled muscle reaction and for nerve impulses to reach and cross the neuromuscular junction. This is very important in cardiac muscle where myocardial contractility depends upon the rapid passage of impulses throughout the heart, and the autonomic nervous system exercises a continuous control.

Treatment

The prime consideration in the treatment of hypoparathyroidism is to raise the plasma calcium and maintain it at a normal level. Unlike some endocrine disorders hormones cannot be given effectively as replacement therapy. Parathyroid hormone is an expensive drug and is difficult to obtain. It is unfortunate that the body, after a short while, develops antibodies against the drug rendering it ineffective. Thus the patient will be given treatment to raise the blood calcium with vitamin D preparations and supplementary calcium, both of which may be taken by mouth. Small amounts of vitamin D are given to begin the treatment. They are raised gradually to avoid plasma calcium levels rising quickly and putting extra work on the kidneys. Supplementary calcium is given in the form of calcium lactate. If the patient demonstrates cardiac disorders on admission it may be necessary to elevate the plasma calcium level quickly. Intravenous infusion of calcium gluconate is one effective method. When the acute phase is passed this can be changed to oral calcium.

Because of the inverse proportion effect on calcium and phosphorus the low level of calcium would indicate a high level of phosphorus. Efforts are needed to reduce the intake of phosphorus and lessen the work of the kidneys in excreting any excess when the calcium level rises. As these two minerals are often found in the same type of foods restriction is made on calcium rich food in the diet. This may appear strange as a high calcium content meal would seem the natural diet to give this patient, however the high phosphorus fraction that accompanies it can cause problems. Such a diet would avoid fish, liver and dairy produce.

Once an acceptable level of plasma calcium has been reached the patient may be discharged from hospital. Aftercare includes regular assessment of the calcium balance. A few hypoparathyroid patients make a spontaneous recovery during their course of treatment when the PTH level returns to normal without assistance. In such cases treatment may be relaxed although regular observation is still necessary. All other patients rely on artificial methods of maintaining their plasma calcium level and here too regular checks are needed to avoid return of hypoparathyroid symptoms.

4
The Pancreas

Experience in hospitals shows that certain disorders may be associated with specific times of the year; an example is gastro-intestinal tract infection which is more prevalent during summer months when the slightest neglect of food hygiene can lead to disasterous results. One such seasonal association relates to the days immediately after Christmas. A patient may be admitted to an acute medical ward, possibly unconscious. The nurse will notice the deep sighing respirations, a rapid pulse, low blood pressure and signs of dehydration. The patient may be of either sex and in no specific age group. When a history is taken it is found that the patient has been attending a hospital outpatient clinic for several years and is usually meticulous about the times, quantities and types of food eaten. Because of the festive season he has been a little careless during the previous few days, including his intake of alcohol and the regularity of the injections he gives himself. The patient is in a coma, a serious complication of the disease diabetes mellitus, an endocrine disorder of the pancreas.

The pancreas is a long organ, often described as 'hammer shaped'. It lies in the curve of the duodenum, behind the stomach, in a transverse position. The head lies in the duodenal curve and is attached to the common bile duct by the pancreatic duct. The middle, or body, lies

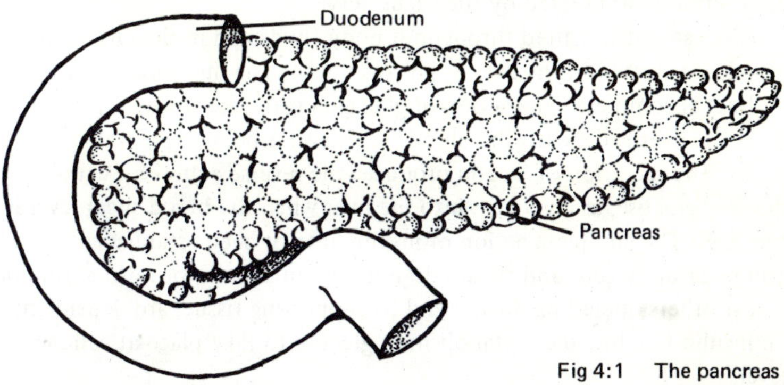

Fig 4:1 The pancreas

across the abdominal aorta and the lumbar vertebrae. The distal end, or tail, lies to the left side and stretches almost to the spleen. The organ contains an abundant supply of nerves and blood vessels lying in the connective tissue of the gland.

The pancreas is a gland having two distinct and separate functions. It is involved in the digestion of food in the alimentary tract, and it produces two hormones concerned with the metabolism of some digestive products. The secretions of the pancreas are:

1 Exocrine secretion which leaves the gland through the pancreatic duct and is composed of pancreatic juice or enzymes of digestion.
2 Endocrine secretion which is absorbed directly into the blood stream and consists of two hormones, insulin and glucagon.

The endocrine secretions of the pancreas are produced in groups of cells scattered throughout the gland. It has been estimated that two million of these cells are present in the normal adult pancreas. They are called the Islets of Langerhan's, or pancreatic islets. The cells are of two distinct types, the alpha cells, forming the minority, and secreting the hormone glucagon and the beta cells secreting the hormone insulin. The action of pancreatic hormones is a continuous process for they are not secreted only when required, but are always present in the circulation in minimal amounts. Secretion varies according to the demand made by the concentration of glucose in the blood passing through the pancreas. This action is stimulated by the vagus nerve.

Glucose is distributed throughout body fluids and in the circulating blood. It is stored in the liver as glycogen when the digestion of carbohydrate is complete. The action of glucagon is to free stored glycogen from the liver cells when the blood sugar level is below acceptable limits. The secretion of insulin produces the reverse action by withdrawing glucose, as glycogen, into the liver when the blood sugar level is too high. The complete action of insulin has not been established. Certain groups of body cells and tissues do not rely on insulin for normal function whilst others, including muscle and its supporting tissue, are dependent on insulin to allow the metabolism of glucose to take place at cellular level.

Although it functions independently the action of this gland cannot be viewed in isolation when considering its effect on blood sugar for other endocrine glands also play a role in the regulation of sugar levels. The thyroid gland may vary the balance of blood sugar by changes in metabolism at cellular level and the adrenal cortex secretes a hormone in the glucocorticoid group that inhibits the breakdown of glucose.

The disorder created by a disturbance of the pancreatic islets is diabetes mellitus, resulting from undersecretion or complete absence of insulin. Because of the inverse effect between insulin and blood sugar the absence of insulin results in an uncontrolled increase in circulating sugars, due to this lack of the natural chemical stabiliser. Such a rise is called hyperglycaemia; the opposite condition, an abnormally low level of blood sugar, being called hypoglycaemia. Many years ago a patient suffering from diabetes mellitus could be expected to live for a limited time only. It was inevitable that he would eventually pass into a coma and die due to ignorance of the causative factors and the lack of efficient treatment. This was the picture until about fifty years ago when two brilliant biochemists isolated the hormone insulin. Since then understanding of the disorder and methods of treatment have made great advances.

The disease is not confined specifically to either sex although the ratio is higher for males in the younger age group. The menopause and pregnancy account for large numbers of female patients. The average age when development of this disorder becomes significant is over fifty years and the numbers increase proportionately with a rise in age above this point. Statistics show that only two patients in every ten are below this critical level of the sixth decade.

Heredity factors are not conclusive although the incidence in younger age groups suggests possible genetic inheritance. Twenty-five per cent. give the history of one blood relation suffering from the disease.

A number of patients are overweight, particularly in the older age group. Although there is no direct connection between diabetes mellitus and obesity, it is considered that overactivity of the pancreatic islets may be the cause, due to excessive intake of carbohydrate.

One obvious cause of diabetes is the surgical removal of the pancreas. The operation of pancreatectomy may be performed if the organ is

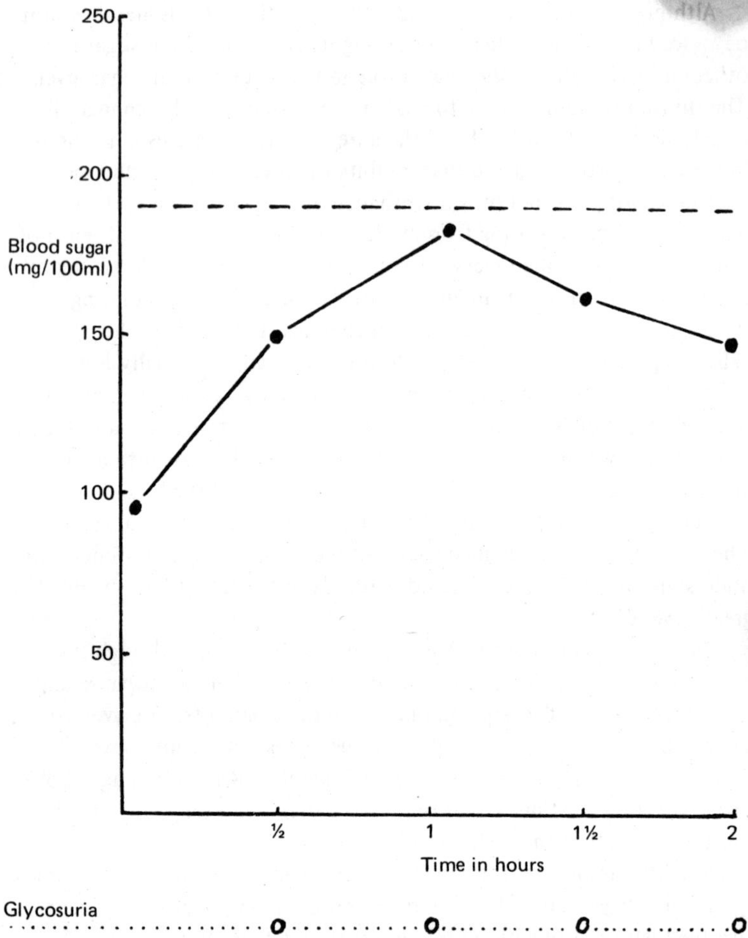

Fig 4:2 The normal curve

severely diseased or is the site of a tumour. In such patients replacement treatment must be started immediately following surgery.

Diabetes mellitus can be defined as a state of incomplete carbohydrate metabolism, due to the lack of adequate insulin. When carbohydrate has been absorbed from the alimentary tract in the form of glucose the lack of insulin impairs its utilisation at tissue and cellular level. Associated with this is the failure of any excess glucose to be converted and stored in the liver. Because of these two abnormalities the blood sugar level is high. Normal readings vary between 60 and 120mg in every 100ml of blood, according to the time the sample is taken after a meal containing carbohydrate has been eaten. When a specimen is taken just before a meal the result will be nearer the lower level and after a meal the blood sugar level quickly reaches its peak.

In uncontrolled diabetes the lack of insulin creates a constant state of hyperglycaemia. The kidney tubules are unable successfully to retain the increased glucose resulting in part of the excess being passed in the urine (glycosuria). From the metabolic breakdown of fatty acids in the liver some products are released into the blood stream to provide energy in muscle tissue, included in these fractions is acetoacetic acid. Because a lack of insulin impairs metabolism at cell level the normally low level of fatty acid fractions are raised resulting in ketones being passed in the urine.

Diabetes mellitus presents a number of diagnostic symptoms. The first may be an excessive output of urine, which is associated with the need to dilute the sugar passing through the kidney. The increased fluid loss will cause the patient to complain of a greater need to drink. The passage of sugar may cause pruritis to develop and this can be complicated by mild infection due to the fact that organisms will flourish in a sugary medium. A loss of weight may be experienced by diabetic patients. Complaints of weakness and of easily becoming tired are also common symptoms.

A primary diagnosis can be made by testing the patient's urine; although not conclusive the presence of sugar and ketones is a firm indication that diabetes may have developed. Simple methods of testing urine to detect these fractions have been devised.

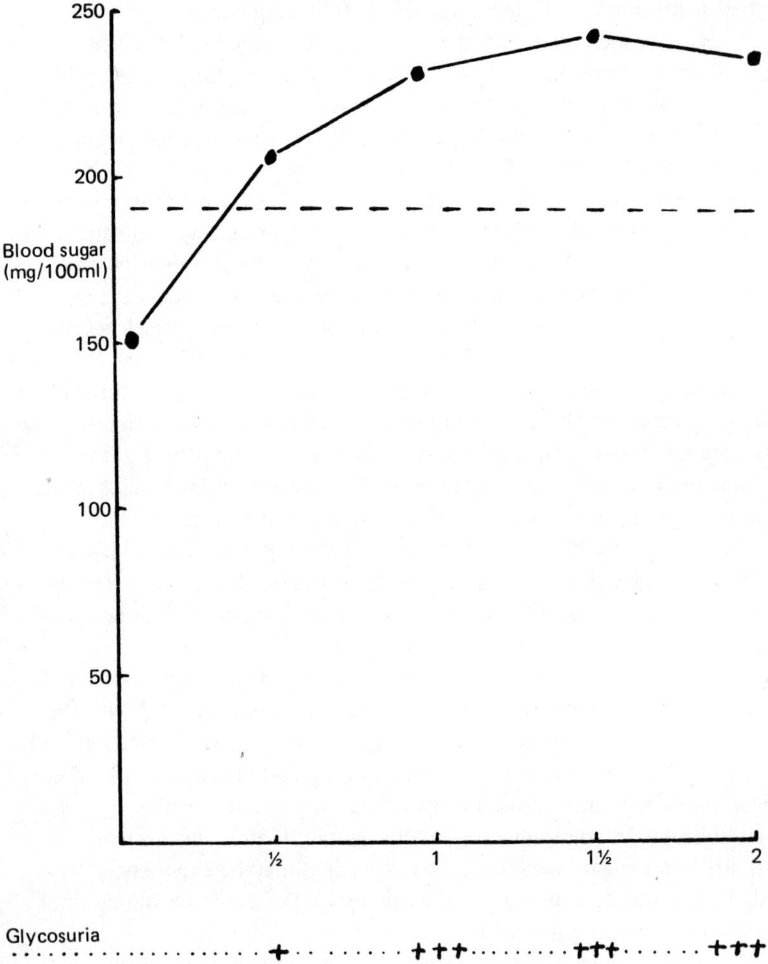

Fig 4:3 The diabetic curve

Methods of testing for sugar

Classic methods of testing for sugar include Fehling's test and Benedict's test, the latter uses a solution containing sodium and copper sulphate. The urine and the solution are mixed in set proportions and boiled in a test tube, the colour changes are indicative of the presence of sugar. These tests have now been replaced by simpler, quicker methods that involve no heating and eliminate the chance of injury from boiling liquids that have a tendency to erupt from test tubes.

A CLINISTIX strip (Ames Company) is a quick test to determine the presence of glucose in urine. It is a narrow plastic strip with a cellulose reagent portion containing chemicals that react to give a colour change when dipped in urine containing glucose. It does not indicate quantity but is a positive or negative indication of glycosuria. In adults, if glycosuria is found CLINITEST (Ames Company) are used to obtain a semi-quantitative reading in the specimen. In young children the CLINITEST tablet should be used first and positive specimens tested with CLINISTIX strips to see if the reducing substance is glucose or some other reducing fraction e.g. galactose.

The CLINITEST tablet is placed in the test tube provided with the exact amount of urine and water recommended. The tablets are self boiling and colour changes are measured against a chart supplied for this purpose.

Methods of testing for ketones

Tests for ketonuria include Rothera's test, requiring a number of chemicals to be added to urine in carefully measured proportions. The method is slow and takes time to prepare but the results are accurate if performed correctly.

Modern methods include KETOSTIX strips (Ames Company), these are plastic strips like clinistix to be dipped into the specimen. Colour changes indicate the presence of ketones and variations of colour also aid in roughly assessing the concentration. An alternative test is the ACETEST tablet (Ames Company). One drop of urine is placed on the tablet with a dropper and the resulting colour indicates the presence, and approximately the concentration, of ketones. Both these tests involve the use of sodium nitro-prusside; they are safe, reliable and quick to perform.

Modern methods of urinalysis are quick and satisfactory but it is necessary to adhere strictly to the instructions, particularly the timing of readings. They must be stored correctly and not contaminated by handling with the fingers.

It is at this point that the nurse will first see the patient who has been admitted for further investigations, diagnosis and treatment. The patient will be admitted to a medical ward following the primary diagnosis, emergency admissions are not the usual mode of entry unless complications occur.

The patient will be told of the reason for entering hospital before admission and therefore will be anxious and apprehensive regarding his health and the outcome of the disease. It is important that on admission any nurses caring for the patient should understand the problems and be prepared to alleviate the immediate stress. It should be explained to the patient that admission to hospital is to confirm the diagnosis and, if necessary, begin a prescribed method of treatment to ensure a quick return to his family and a normal life. It is important that the patient realises it is not a disorder causing him to be permanently incapacitated and it is at this time particularly that the nurse plays a part in the patient's recovery by the development of his own confidence.

Physically the patient may reveal no sign of the disease when first seen. Because of the complications that can develop care and observation of the patient's skin, particularly when bathing, are necessary. Major problems can be avoided if skin lesions are noticed early and treated. Metabolic changes cause the skin to heal slowly therefore patients who remain in bed, especially the elderly, require regular skin care to ensure that pressure areas do not break down. Women in the older age group often suffer from pruritis vulvae. The constant soreness and itching of the external genitalia leads to scratching which may cause a painful rash if allowed to continue untreated. A similar condition can develop in men with soreness and itching on and around the scrotum. Patients suffering from pruritis are acutely embarrassed and may tolerate the discomfort for a long time rather than call the nurse's attention to it. This is bad for the patient both physically and psychologically. The good nurse, who brings imagination as well as knowledge to her task of caring for her patients, will anticipate this embarrassment and make a point of gently asking whether there is any discomfort in this area without waiting for the patient to tell her. When pruritis does occur frequent bathing of the parts is necessary, normal saline or a solution of bicarbonate of soda (one teaspoonful to 500ml of tepid water) is more effective in reducing the soreness than plain water. Soap should be avoided when possible, but an application of soothing cream such as calamine may prove helpful.

Diabetic patients are subject to the development of gangrene in circumstances where the circulation is impaired. In anticipation of such changes it is necessary for regular observations to be carried out of the patient's extremities. If the fingers and toes become discoloured it should be reported immediately for specific treatment. In patients who have suffered with undetected diabetes of long standing a further complication is the appearance of cataract of the eye. The patient may complain of reading difficulties even when wearing their spectacles. Any such complaint is worthy of investigation.

Because of the polyuria the patient will require a larger fluid intake. Younger patients are able to ask when thirsty whilst older and possibly debilitated patients will need assistance to reach a sufficient intake to balance with their output. To ensure a satisfactory fluid regime a fluid balance chart should be used; the patient's intake should equal his output, including insensible losses. The use of such a chart will also serve as an indicator of kidney function, for changes may occur in kidney tissue causing some degree of functional failure.

From admission regular examination of urine specimens is essential. Specimens are collected at four-hourly intervals, tests for sugar and ketones are performed and a careful record of the times and results must be kept. Particular importance is placed on early morning and evening specimens because of the variation in blood sugar after night fasting and following the meals taken during the day. When treatment has commenced regular testing of urine is an indication of the progress made by the patient and will also aid in avoiding the serious complication of coma. The disease diabetes mellitus can produce coma, or loss of consciousness, in two distinct ways; hyperglycaemic coma (see page 76) and hypoglycaemic coma (see page 78).

The admission to hospital of patients suffering with suspected diabetes mellitus will allow assessment of three aspects of the disease.

1 Laboratory confirmation of the disease
2 Regulation of dietary intake
3 Dosage of insulin required

Laboratory test for diabetes mellitus

A glucose tolerance test is designed to assess the patient's metabolism when given oral carbohydrate under controlled conditions. The findings of the laboratory examination provide a graph of blood sugar levels at regular intervals, combined with this are the result of urine tests at the same times to show the points at which glucose filters through the kidney and produces glycosuria (see illustration 4:3).

Preparation of the patient includes an explanation of the procedure, its purpose and the method to be used. The nurse should aim at getting not just a passive obedience from the patient, but his active cooperation. In this instance it should be explained that the test is to confirm the diagnosis made by the patient's own doctor; that it will be necessary to take samples of the patient's blood and urine at regular intervals, and that if the test is to be a success he must not eat or drink anything unless told to do so.

The patient must take nothing by mouth after 9 pm the previous evening allowing the test to commence at 9 am the following morning, thus minimising the time that the patient is deprived of food. At 9 am a specimen of blood is taken to determine the patient's 'fasting' sugar level ie the level of a person who has not eaten for at least four to six hours. In normal subjects the fasting blood sugar is near the minimum level following a fast (60 to 120mg/100ml). The diabetic patient will not have such a low level and a degree of glycosuria is possible. Also at this time the patient is required to empty his bladder, a specimen being retained.

The patient is given 50gm of glucose by mouth. It is usual to mix it with some flavouring in 100ml of water, the result being more palatable. The patient should be at rest from this time and no smoking is allowed. From the time the glucose is given blood specimens are taken every half hour afterwards until four specimens are collected. The patient is required to pass a specimen of urine half hourly during the two hours. The blood specimens need to be collected in bottles containing a preservative, the amount to be collected is marked on the label. Care is necessary to ensure that each bottle is marked with the patient's name and the time collected. When specimens are collected they should be marked immediately to avoid mistakes. Careless marking or timing can result in a faulty graph and cause repetition of the procedure with added stress to the patient. All specimens are dispatched to the laboratory as soon as possible while the samples are fresh.

The result of the test is received in the form of a graph showing an estimation of blood sugar levels coupled with urinalysis. The curve of a normal subject starts at a lower level that the diabetic patient and will rise quickly during the first half hour, insulin then controls the blood sugar level by withdrawing any excess. Glycosuria will be negative in each specimen.

The curve of the diabetic patient starts at a much higher point in the scale and it quickly rises during the first half hour and then continues to rise at a slower rate. The fall of blood sugar does not reach the fasting reading until several hours have passed. Glycosuria may be positive from the first sample or during the first hour. Minor degrees of diabetes may be impossible to diagnose until the test for glucose tolerance is performed. Once confirmed treatment should begin as soon as possible.

Regulation of diet

Insulin is destroyed by products of the gastro-intestinal tract, a property shared by most endocrine secretions. Therefore any insulin given therapeutically must be given by injection. Normally the pancreas secretes insulin according to the body's needs. As the diabetic patient cannot vary his insulin level, except at the time of injection, stabilisation and balance is partly controlled by the intake of carbohydrate. To enable this to be done treatment is directed at estimating the quantity of food, particularly carbohydrate, required by the patient in his daily needs. The calorific value of the food is then equated with the amount of insulin necessary to maintain the blood sugar within safe limits throughout twenty-four hours.

It is difficult to produce rules for this balanced diet, each individual performs a variety of tasks in their daily life. Some occupations are strenuous and demand a large output of energy while others with more sedentary jobs need much less. Other factors that influence the calorific need include the body size and the age of the patient, a growing child will need more Calories than a tiny elderly person who has retired from active life. Tables have been designed on which a basis of dietary need can be estimated. The quantity of insulin required to balance this food can be assessed according to the patient's own production of insulin and the levels of blood sugar demonstrated through a twenty-four hour span. The diet is arranged to give a constant amount of carbohydrate each day, by regular tests adjustments are made until the ideal amount is achieved.

Insulin

The hormone insulin is a complex protein molecule. Following its discovery patients were treated with pancreatic extractions in a crude form derived from animals, a method that left much to be desired as the amount given was difficult to control and the substance rather unpalatable. Today insulin is given by subcutaneous injection. It is supplied in rubber capped 10ml bottles and is calibrated in units. The solution is prepared in three strengths, twenty units per ml (single strength), forty units per ml (double strength) and eighty units per ml (quadruple strength). By using a suitable strength the patient can receive the appropriate number of units in the smallest volume thus reducing the size of the injection. When prescribing insulin consideration is given to the time taken before the hormone becomes effective and the duration of its activity. To assist in this control there are two main divisions of insulin available, quick acting and slow acting.

Soluble insulin

This is a clear solution, quick acting but of short duration. It is ideal for new patients where insulin needs have not been established. Soluble insulin acts quickly reaching its maximum effect after three hours but loses its activity two to three hours later. Because of this quick action it is necessary for the patient to receive two injections daily.

Zinc suspension insulin

Zinc suspension insulin is produced in several forms that differ in the time taken for the hormone to become active and in the length of activity. The difference is created by precipitation of insulin into zinc crystals, the size of the molecule varies the absorption rate when taken into the blood stream.

Semilente

Consisting of fine particles that have a maximum effect after eight hours and end after twelve hours.

Lente

Becomes active after two to three hours reaching a maximum action after ten hours and a duration of activity of approximately twenty-four hours.

Ultralente

A very slow acting insulin, does not reach its maximum effect for about eighteen hours and has a duration of twenty-four to thirty-six hours.

Other types of insulin are available, their action is within the range of soluble and the zinc suspensions. Soluble insulin is made in all three strengths other types are only prepared in double and quadruple strengths.

Insulin is administered with a special syringe calibrated in units for ease of measurement and to reduce the chance of mistakes when a patient prepares their own injection. It is important to remember that the procedure of giving insulin by injection is not only performed by nurses, for the patient will continue to inject himself when discharged from hospital. To reduce further the chance of accident insulin is packaged with different coloured labels on the cartons and bottles according to the strength and type to enable the patient to identify the correct bottle before use.

Oral hypoglycaemic agents

Oral hypoglycaemic agents are often prescribed for diabetic patients in the older age group. Insulin is destroyed in the presence of gastric secretions, so the drugs taken by mouth are not insulin but are compounds designed to stimulate a supply of insulin from the pancreas of the patient. There are two groups of oral hypoglycaemic agents.

Sulphonureas
Preparations in this group are thought to stimulate the beta cells of the pancreas to promote insulin secretion. Tolbutamide is one agent in this group, which is quickly excreted and requires to be taken twice daily for complete regulation of blood sugar. Chlorpropamide on the other hand is excreted at a much slower rate and can be effectively administered as one single daily dose.

Biguanides
The drugs in the biguanide group do not stimulate the pancreatic islets although the presence of insulin is necessary before they are activated. They are thought to have a direct effect on the metabolism of glucose in the tissues. Phenformin is one example of this group.

Treatment

It has been estimated that approximately thirty per cent. of all new cases of confirmed diabetes mellitus can be controlled by diet alone, the remainder need either a combination of diet and oral hypoglycaemic agents or diet and insulin. It can be readily understood from these statistics that all diabetic patients need some form of dietary control. Diet supervision is necessary for three reasons.

1 To reduce the weight of the patient, obesity often being a cause of diabetic symptoms.
2 To control diabetes of the milder type, possibly with the assistance of oral hypoglycaemic agents.
3 To control the disorder in conjunction with insulin.

Reducing the weight of the patient

Insulin production is often sufficient to meet the needs of a normal body mass but the pancreas cannot secrete the extra necessary to compensate for the added bulk of obesity. To reduce weight the patient will be given a diet as low as 800–1,000 Calories each day, in controlled conditions with regular observation. When the weight is reduced the effect is noticeable by the disappearance of glycosuria. If glycosuria continues after the patient has reached an acceptable weight it may be necessary to supplement the treatment with oral hypoglycaemic agents.

Control of mild diabetes

In this type of diabetes the patient is not suffering from complete failure of the pancreatic islets but is secreting a limited amount of insulin. Included in this group are the majority of patients who develop diabetes during later life, when it may be due to reduction in numbers of the islets from a diminished blood supply and cellular atrophy. If the patient is to be controlled without drugs it is necessary to reduce his dietary intake of carbohydrate to balance the reduction in insulin

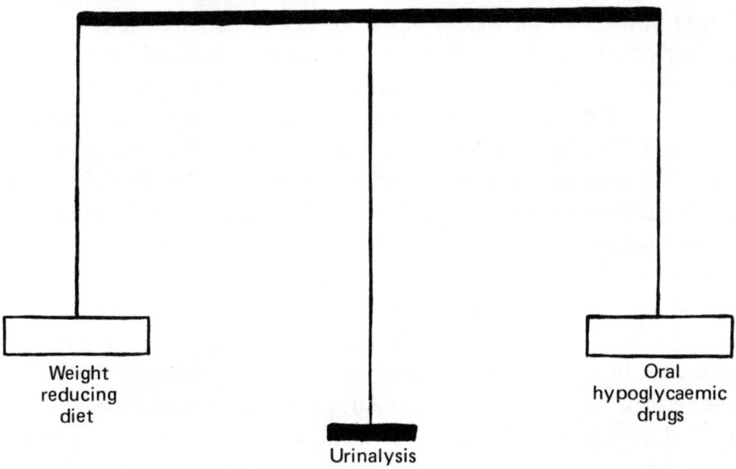

Fig 4:4 Control of mild diabetes

secreted. The amount will vary with each patient, often he can be stabilised by a sensible, well balanced diet having a low carbohydrate content. Estimation of dietary need can be made by regular testing of urine specimens at four hourly intervals. When a balance is reached the ideal specimen will register a minute percentage of sugar, ie a Clinitest specimen will show a change from blue to slightly green. This indicates that the patient's blood sugar is neither high enough to be dangerous or so low as to cause hypoglycaemic complications.

If the urine is constantly registering a high level of sugar when the diet is controlled it may be necessary to supplement the treatment with hypoglycaemic agents. Once a satisfactory therapeutic pattern has been established regular checks are made at hospital outpatient clinics.

Control of diabetes with insulin and diet

Patients receiving insulin therapy are severely deficient in pancreatic hormones. When calculating the dietary and insulin needs of the patient having initial stabilisation it is important to consider the daily energy requirement. The diet is directed towards meeting this energy need and maintaining body weight. The average intake of carbohydrate should contain approximately 150 to 200gms and the meals must be spread throughout the waking day to avoid long periods when the patient's blood sugar may drop below a safe level. It should include one late, easily digested meal before retiring to avoid hypoglycaemia whilst asleep. The distribution of carbohydrate is partly governed by the type of insulin taken by the patient. Using soluble insulin a meal is necessary following the injection to equate with its fast action. Insulins of the lente group allow meals to be spread evenly without such strict relationship to the injection. Control of both insulin and diet is made by regular assessment of fresh urine specimens using tests for sugar and acetone. The ideal balance is reached when urine demonstrates a slight change of colour using Clinitest tablets, indicating that the patient is neither hyper-glycaemic or hypoglycaemic. As a confirmation of urine tests, and to ensure their validity with each patient, checks of the blood sugar are made during the first weeks of treatment. When a satisfactory degree of control between diet and insulin has been reached the patient will be reassessed following a period of time at home in their normal environ-

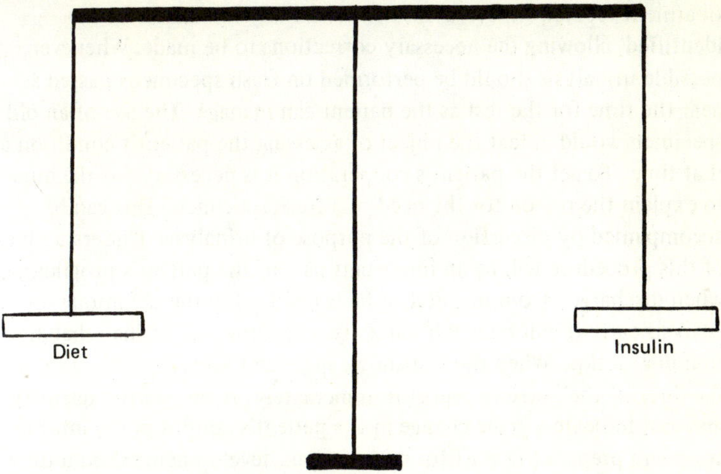

Fig 4:5 Control of severe diabetes

ment and occupation, any adjustments necessary can then be made.

One essential feature of a diabetic diet is the need to encourage the use of a wide variety of foods. Because a diet is prescribed it does not mean that the food eaten should lack variety or be uninteresting. Hospitals caring for diabetic patients offer suggested methods of assessing amounts of a wide variety of foods. Such charts are explained to the patient and given to them when leaving hospital. The amounts may be quoted in grams or in corresponding homely measures such as a teaspoon or teacup. Instructions may also include foods that can be taken in less restricted amounts, such as green vegetables. Special foods are manufactured for diabetic patients with limited carbohydrate contents. Diabetic chocolate and jam are produced with a limited Calorie content stated on the container that must be taken into account when measuring the daily allowance.

The responsibilities of the nurse to the patient during stabilisation are primarily concerned with safety and the avoidance of immediate complications. The objective of reaching a satisfactory balance of diet and insulin, or oral hypoglycaemic agents, is dependent upon accurate recording and observation by the ward staff. From the beginning of treatment regular urinalysis is essential for any imbalance to be identified, allowing the necessary corrections to be made. Whenever possible urinalysis should be performed on fresh specimens passed as near the time for the test as the patient can manage. The use of an old specimen would defeat the object of assessing the patient's condition at that time. To get the patient's cooperation it is necessary for the nurse to explain the reason for the need of a fresh specimen. This can be accompanied by discussion of the purpose of urinalysis. Understanding of this procedure will be an important part of the patient's programme when discharged from hospital. If he is involved in the technique of analysis early it will reduce his anxiety and form part of the rehabilitation instruction. When the test shows sugar and acetone fractions it is the duty of the nurse to report it immediately. Although the quantity may not indicate a grave change in the patient's condition the information will prepare the staff for more serious developments should they arise and it will show the need for strict observation. It may cause the patient some concern that he is receiving more specific attention than before, so to allay these fears the reason can be explained in simple terms.

During the preliminary stages of treatment it is inevitable that some degree of imbalance will develop as the need for every patient is different and cannot be accurately related to another. Although approximate calculations can be made the possibility of complications must be considered until the physician is satisfied that a state of equilibrium is reached and coma is no longer a hazard.

Hyperglycaemic coma

Hyperglycaemic coma, also called diabetic coma, is the more serious of these extremes. Because the onset is gradual the patient may not be able to inform the ward staff he is not feeling well. A typical sign first noticed by the observant nurse is the patient's breathing for he may display signs of 'air hunger', gasping with the mouth open and showing noticeable chest movements. When approached there is a peculiar smell on his breath, an odour often described as new mown hay, which is an early indication of circulating acetone. This can be anticipated and a watch made if the patient complains of a loss of appetite, slight vomiting or abdominal pain and nausea during the preceding hours. Good nursing observation will suspect the impending signs of a developing coma, and an immediate report should be made. The suspicion can be confirmed by testing a specimen of urine taken at that time when sugar and acetone will be found. The physician may order soluble insulin to be given and glucose by mouth if possible, otherwise an intravenous infusion will be necessary. Glucose is given to prevent a rapid reversal of the hyperglycaemia when the insulin becomes active; it is at this point that the glucose balance is critical and too much insulin may cause hypoglycaemia. Because of the urgency of the situation it may be necessary to pass a catheter if a specimen of urine is not passed freely by the patient. This procedure will be ordered by the physician and should not be undertaken without his consent. The indiscriminate passing of catheters is a practice to be avoided and should only be used in an emergency, particularly where the patient's risk of sepsis is increased due to poor resistance. If necessary, the procedure must be carried out using the utmost care to reduce the chance of urinary infection.

If the patient is unconscious an intravenous infusion will be necessary as this allows continuous treatment to prevent dehydration and provides a route for administration of insulin and glucose. This is a critical period for the patient and the responsibilities of the nurse are greatly increased. Careful testing of all specimens of urine is needed, often the result of these will be a deciding factor in any variation of treatment. The hazard of caring for an unconscious patient is complicated by loss of body fluids, as this creates the possibility of the mouth becoming very dry. Frequent attention is necessary to maintain the skin and prevent pressure sores, bed bathing should be carried out at least once daily and special care is given to pressure areas at regular intervals. The patient is turned when possible to reduce pressure and friction, such movements are limited however due to the infusion which must be maintained.

It is necessary to use extra care when dealing with the mouth of an unconscious patient. Oral toilet is an important part of nursing treatment but caution is needed to prevent material used in the procedure from entering the respiratory tract The cough reflex is missing in this patient and respiratory infection will develop from inhaled substances.

When the patient regains consciousness the physician will adjust the insulin and diet to regain stability. It is important that all nurses know of such changes as the incorrect measurement of diet or insulin will result in delay to the patient's recovery. Diet received from the kitchen will be measured and prepared when sent to the ward. It is usual to send such diets in containers to eliminate mistakes, the patient's name being attached to the container. The timing of meals is important, remembering the correlation between food and insulin. The patient must eat all the food provided at each meal and if he declines to eat the full meal substitutions will be necessary.

Hypoglycaemic coma

Hypoglycaemic coma presents a different picture for here the patient has an abnormally low blood sugar level. The onset of the coma is sudden, the tongue and lips tingle, the patient becomes anxious followed by confusion and restlessness. Pallor and sweating may develop and the patient becomes drowsy, followed by coma. The most important aspect of treatment is speed and good nursing observations of a patient during stabilisation will prevent the condition developing to a dangerous level. As the low blood sugar is the cause of this complication it is vital that glucose is administered quickly once the diagnosis is confirmed. Treatment is directed at elevation of the patient's blood sugar and oral glucose should be given when possible. But if the patient is unconscious there are three methods by which this may be done.

1 Glucose can be given through an intravenous injection.
2 Glucose may be given via a naso-gastric tube passed into the stomach. Care must be exercised in passing the tube as the patient possesses no cough reflex to warn the nurse of entry into the trachea.
3 The patient may be given an injection of glucagon, this frees glycogen from the liver and in an emergency can be sufficient to allow the patient to regain consciousness and continue with oral treatment.

If patients are made aware of the warning signs of hypoglycaemic coma the chance of this grave condition developing when discharged from hospital are reduced. It is therefore desirable that patients should have personal experience of hypoglycaemia, and how to deal with it, before leaving hospital. The symptoms may vary from one person to another and a description is insufficient for a condition which, when it occurs, may render him helpless before he understands what is happening to him. A more practical approach is to allow him, under the constant observation of an experienced nurse, to become hypoglycaemic. He will then be aware of his own symptom pattern and the dramatic reversal of the symptoms which takes place when he eats a few lumps of sugar. Such a patient will face the future with more confidence and will be better equipped to care for himself than one who has only listened to a description from a nurse or doctor. He should also appreciate that most hypoglycaemic attacks are caused by, too much insulin, too little food or too much exercise, and that he must bear these factors in mind when planning his daily activities.

Once stabilisation has been established the patient can return home and resume a normal, but organised, life. Because of the initial problems encountered during his stay in hospital he may feel very apprehensive about undertaking his own treatment and observations. The worry of this responsibility with no one to check his progress can cause the patient some concern. The ward nurse plays a major role in allaying these fears during the rehabilitation of the diabetic. During the period before discharge from hospital the patient will be instructed in the art of urine testing and the method of recording his findings, with emphasis on the significance of each change of colour. He is also shown the method of calculating doses and drawing up insulin into the special syringe designed for this purpose. To nurses with experience in such procedures the techniques may appear rather elementary, but to the patient this is a new and important venture designed to offer him the chance to live an uncomplicated life in the future. The patient may find difficulty in performing these tasks and think he has not acquired a sufficient degree of skill to manage, particularly if he is in the older age group, some of whom do not grasp ideas quickly. To support the patient at this time the nurse should accompany him, checking the results and pointing out any errors that occur. When the patient is able to carry out the procedures unaided a nurse should always be ready to check the patient's results when asked. This is particularly important in the case of insulin drawn into a syringe where a mistake can be dangerous. The patient will need instruction in the technique of insulin injections, including care of syringes and needles. They should be boiled each week and stored between injections in a special container of spirit, being rinsed in boiled water before and after use and examined occasionally to ensure the syringe plunger is not leaking. Sites for injection must be discussed and the necessity of varying the site regularly; the areas used are the abdominal wall, the front and outer aspect of the thighs and the upper arm. The injection technique is important and some encouragement is necessary before the patient is proficient and able to manage unaided.

The importance of diet should be stressed to a patient commencing a diabetic routine. Because it seems of greater significance the patient will be meticulous about insulin injections and urinalysis and the balance of food may not have the same impact as it is an everyday part of his life. If the need for careful selection and measurement is shown constantly he will approach the problem with more care when food is prepared by himself or his family.

He should be instructed in the extra care needed with personal hygiene with emphasis on care of the feet and toenails to prevent sepsis. This should include reasonable trimming of toenails frequently. The patient will be advised to seek his doctor's help in cases of illness or emergency when he cannot follow his treatment schedule, and provided with a card stating he is a diabetic patient, his name and address and that of his medical practitioner. He is told to carry the card with him at all times. Finally he should always carry sugar, in lump form, in his pocket in case of hypoglycaemic symptoms.

Complications of diabetes mellitus

Among the complications of diabetes only two have been mentioned, hypoglycaemic and hyperglycaemic coma. Because blood affects almost all body tissues changes can take place in many sites so two of the more common problems are included here.

Cardiovascular changes

Hardening of the arteries (arteriosclerosis) can occur at an earlier age in diabetic patients, particularly in the peripheral vessels of the limbs. Because of the diminished blood supply there is a risk of gangrene. Normal healing is also retarded. Men in particular may disregard small cuts and abrasions sustained at work unless the danger of neglect is clearly explained to them. The problem is not only one of poor healing but also of reduced natural body defence to the entry of pathogenic organisms. Arterial changes also create a greater chance of coronary thrombosis in the young diabetic patient.

Infection

Diabetic patients are prone to minor infections of the skin, including boils. This is noticeable when blood sugar is not controlled and can be the first sign that takes the patient to the doctor who makes the primary diagnosis. They are also more susceptible to chest infections including pulmonary tuberculosis.

Diabetes and surgery

Although diabetic patients are more liable to develop disorders that require surgical treatment as the result of cardiovascular changes eg gangrene, they are also subject to the normal disorders needing surgical intervention. The major problem is the change in metabolism produced by the procedure including the effect of anaesthetic together with the added chance of sepsis and reduced healing. Surgery on diabetic patients may be considered in two groups.

Emergency cases

Patients admitted in need of immediate surgery, such as appendicitis or perforated gastric ulcer, warrant special consideration for the condition of the patient on admission is of paramount importance. If the emergency has caused an upset of his diabetic routine the patient may be dehydrated and in need of stabilisation. This can be precipitated by neglect of his diet and insulin injections with further aggravation if sepsis is involved. In such a patient it is necessary to achieve a degree of stability during treatment of the surgical condition. An intravenous infusion provides a means of reducing dehydration and a route for the administration of insulin and glucose. While the patient is anaesthetised the blood sugar level is maintained within acceptable limits by taking blood samples at regular intervals and administering soluble insulin and glucose through the infusion.

Waiting list cases

Patients entering hospital for surgery without the stress of emergency can be considered for careful pre-operative preparation. Insulin may be changed from the slow acting group to soluble, allowing rapid variation according to the patient's need. Careful balance of the diet is necessary to keep the patient in good physical condition for the operation. The problem of starving the patient during the hours before surgery is partly overcome by drinking flavoured glucose fluids up to three hours before operation. This gives stability until the operation begins when blood sugar is controlled by laboratory tests.

General post-operative care

In both routine and emergency surgery the post-operative care is concentrated on stabilisation. During the immediate hours following operation the patient may be unable to take fluids by mouth and equilibrium is maintained through the infusion. An important nursing responsibility is regular, accurate recording of each urine specimen for it is on the result of these tests that insulin and Calorie equivalents are based. When the patient has passed the immediate post-operative phase and is able to take diet by mouth a routine will commence to re-establish permanent stabilisation.

Post-operative nursing of the diabetic patient involves special features that have an important bearing on his recovery. During the time that he remains in bed particular note should be made of his pressure areas. If reddening of the skin is seen it will be necessary to turn him more frequently. Early ambulation is important. As the extremities may suffer impairment of the circulation regular passive exercises are needed until the patient is able to walk and exercise himself. To allow uncomplicated healing all aseptic procedures should be performed with extreme care. Elimination of infection in a wound is the ideal for any surgery, the need in diabetic patients is greater due to their lower resistance to infection. Should infection be suspected or healing delayed it must be reported immediately to allow a check for organisms and possible antibiotic therapy.

Diabetes and pregnancy

It is possible for diabetes mellitus to exist in a latent form which only becomes apparent when the sufferer is subject to certain forms of stress including infection, surgery or pregnancy. Although the risk of diabetes in acute infection or surgery presents difficulties the condition can be corrected during treatment with little danger to the patient. The development of diabetes during pregnancy does carry extra problems, not only to the mother but also to the foetus. Statistics show that less than one percent of the population are known diabetic sufferers, so it has been assumed that a number of people are sub-clinical diabetics showing little or no evidence. This number corresponds with ante-natal figures which show that one patient in four hundred develops diabetic symptoms during her pregnancy. To reduce the chance of the undiscovered diabetic continuing pregnancy without treatment urine tests for glycosuria are carried out at visits to ante-natal clinics. If urinalysis is positive for sugar further investigations are necessary to confirm the diagnosis. If diabetes develops during pregnancy it is likely to be during the first six months which is a crucial period for the foetus.

Although there appears to be no increase in maternal mortality from diabetes during pregnancy it does have a pronounced effect on the child. All diabetic patients ideally should be admitted by the thirty-second week as this allows continuous observation. Following the puerperium an assessment of the diabetes is made. Often patients who have developed the disorder during pregnancy will be free of glycosuria after parturition. Those who continue to demonstrate clinical signs will require reassessment with a view to long term treatment. Observations of the child must be made at regular intervals to ensure that it has suffered no effects from the mother's disorder.

A large number of neonatal deaths are attributed to respiratory failure. This has been related to a reduction in uterine contractions and a prolonged labour. Because of this physiological change it is often thought advisable to induce premature labour on or about the thirty-seventh week and in certain cases Caesarian section is used. The cause of intra-uterine death is not clearly understood, the numbers vary according to the degree of diabetes; but hyperglycaemic and hypoglycaemic states are contributing factors. There is also a tendency for large amounts of amniotic fluid (hydrammios) to develop. The growth of the foetus in an environment with high blood sugar levels usually causes them to be larger than normal.

The patient who develops the disease before pregnancy will be stabilised and only require adjustment in her insulin and Calorie intake. The patient who is diagnosed after pregnancy has started will need primary stabilisation to avoid complications. Regular assessments are necessary to maintain a normal blood sugar.

Diabetes in children

Diabetes is less common in children than in adults but when it does occur it is usually severe and needs insulin with controlled diet. Because of the difficulty in stabilising children it is often referred to as 'brittle' diabetes. Problems arise in the dietary routine of children due to the variation in their need for energy giving foods. This relates to exercise and the increased needs of the body when growing. There is also the difficulty of children being given food they may dislike which they leave unfinished. Because of these problems it is not easy to stabilise children on a regular amount of insulin and careful observations are needed to prevent development of coma. Often they require more insulin in the initial stages after which the child's ability to produce more insulin naturally may increase as they grow.

Nurses play a major part in the education of the diabetic child as they are able to relieve the obvious anxiety that will be present when treatment first begins. Depending on the age of the child he may be aware of the importance of the disorder and of the need for care when he is discharged from hospital. Support at this time may be vital to the child's future understanding of his problems and in the development of the correct attitude that the disease is not a severe handicap for a normal life is perfectly possible.

One important aspect of diabetes in children is the attitude that needs to be developed in the parents of the child. It is important that they realise the precise nature of their child's disease and the needs of the child. When discharged from hospital it is the parent's responsibility to ensure that the correct pattern of treatment is followed and that it will need to be supervised by them. They will need to give support and encouragement to the child to carry out his own treatment. To enable this positive attitude to be developed the parents can be guided by the medical and nursing staff of the ward who will need to show them the method of measuring and administering insulin correctly, estimating diets and performing urinalysis. The nurse, because of her intimate contact with the patient, can instil into both the patient and the parents the importance of working together to maintain the treatment routine. She can also offer advice on problems that can arise and their prevention, particularly with regard to signs of coma. Parental observation can be valuable for the less obvious complications such as the appearance of the child's skin when bathing; complaints of difficult vision; rashes that may be covered by clothing; itching and local inflammation. The need to look for these changes should be stressed, coupled with an emphasis of the importance of reporting such signs to their own doctor for his advice. Children do not feel as apprehensive and disabled as adults imagine, unless their nurses and parents make them feel so. Even very young children will learn to measure insulin and give themselves injections, often with less shrinking than adults, provided – and this is important – the nurse adopts the right attitude from the start that this is an interesting and important thing to do, and praises the child generously for every advance in technique.

When he returns home his parents must try in every way possible to let him do what other children are doing, even at the slight risk of complications on occasions. He will have this disability all of his life and he needs to learn what he can and cannot do to adjust to his disorder. To make him dependent on others can cause problems in later life. The parents need as much, if not more, support and guidance than the child because their attitude is so important in his rehabilitation. If this relationship between parent and child is made, initially by the doctor and reinforced by the nursing staff, the chance of future difficulties will be reduced.

Hyperinsulinism

Instances of hyperinsulinism are occasionally diagnosed. These patients have the reverse condition to that found in diabetes mellitus. Instead of high blood sugar levels the patient is subject to spontaneous hypoglycaemic states. This phenomenon is caused by increased insulin secretion. One cause is a tumour involving the beta cells (insulinoma), which may pass unnoticed due to difficulty of diagnosis and the rarity of the disorder. Treatment is by surgical intervention for removal of the tumour. Other causes of hyperinsulinism include excessive nervous stimulation by the vagus nerve. This is associated with persons of a nervous disposition and may be transient in its effect requiring no specific care or treatment.

5

Adrenal Gland

Patients coming into hospital are forced to make major adjustments to their way of life. They are surrounded by strange faces in unnatural circumstances and with the loss of the privacy of their own home. It is important that in making these adjustments the patient does not lose his self respect. By treating him with kindness and consideration the nurse can do much to make this potentially impersonal environment more welcoming.

Even in the ideal circumstances some patients can never be as comfortable as others. There are many reasons for this not the least of which is the problem of physical abnormalities causing the person to be acutely self conscious in the close proximity of others. An example is the woman with a masculine appearance. Such a person would be aware of her manly build, her hairy arms and legs and of the obvious growth of hair on her chin and upper lip. Hidden beneath her clothes she also has an abnormal growth of hair over her chest and abdomen, the thought of which creates her anxiety and discomfort. Such a patient may be suffering with a disorder of the adrenal glands.

The adrenal glands consist of two triangular shaped structures fixed to the upper poles of the kidneys. They lie on the posterior wall of the abdominal cavity and are golden yellow in colour. In cross section they show two distinct parts, the yellow outer layer or cortex, and a dark reddish centre the medulla. Each gland has a rich blood supply arising from the superior, middle and inferior suprarenal arteries. They originate from the abdominal aorta and encircle the gland with a network of arterioles supplying a mass of tiny vessels throughout the gland tissue. The venous return differs in that all the blood is collected and taken through one major vein, the suprarenal vein.

The splanchnic nerves, originating from the spinal cord, supply the adrenal glands. The medulla has a complex nerve supply which controls the dilatation and contraction of blood vessels. The two parts of the gland, cortex and medulla, produce different hormones.

Like other organs of the system the adrenal gland does not work

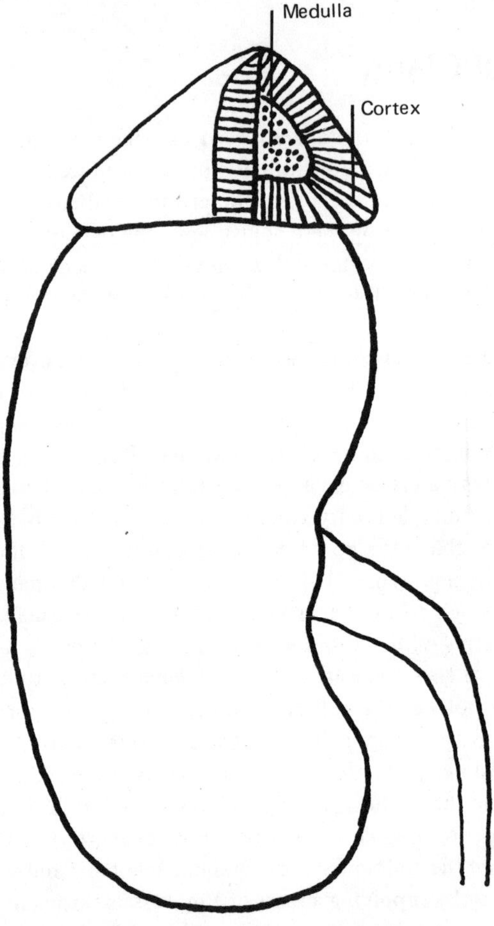

Fig 5:1 The adrenal gland

independently but plays a part in the complex process of metabolism. It has a direct relationship with the anterior pituitary gland which controls all secretions of the cortex, except aldosterone, by the trophic hormone ACTH.

Adrenal cortex

Hormones of the cortex are collectively called steroids. The steroid hormones, of which over forty types have been isolated, fall into three divisions; of this number a few are essential to life.

1 Mineralocorticoids

This group contains a number of hormones that have an effect on mineral balance by controlling the excretion of body minerals through the kidneys. They have a pronounced effect on the kidney tubule by reabsorbing sodium from the glomerular filtrate in exchange for potassium and hydrogen ions. The chief hormone of this group is aldosterone, which differs from other cortical hormones because its secretion is not stimulated by ACTH. The controlling mechanism is not clearly understood although aldosterone is continually secreted in limited amounts to promote the retention of salt and water.

2 Glucocorticoids

These have an effect on the metabolism of carbohydrates and proteins in the body. The major hormones of this group include cortisol and cortisone. Cortisol (hydrocortisone) is the hormone that affects the anterior pituitary lobe to secrete ACTH. The main effect of glucocorticoids in the metabolism of the body is the stimulation of gluconeogenesis (carbohydrate formation) from proteins. If they are present in excess an abnormal loss of nitrogen in the urine may result, leaving the body deficient of protein. Glucocorticoids are antagonistic to insulin and can cause hyperglycaemia and glycosuria when adrenal dysfunction suppresses insulin action.

Glucocorticoids also reduce inflammatory responses of the body. This knowledge has resulted in the therapeutic use of hormones in certain acute disorders.

3 Androgens

Androgens are necessary for the development of secondary sex characteristics, particularly in males, in whom it involves protein synthesis and the increase of muscle mass over the body.

Adrenal medulla

Two hormones are secreted by the adrenal medulla and belong to the group called the catecholamines.

1 Adrenaline

The main functions of adrenaline are to:

a increase oxygen consumption at tissue level
b Stimulate the heart and increase the cardiac output
c Excite and stimulate the nervous system in conditions of stress
d Mobilise liver glycogen and raise the level of blood sugar

2 Noradrenaline

This is similar to adrenaline in composition and its functions include:

a Raising the blood pressure by constricting peripheral blood vessels
b Raising the level of fatty acids in the circulation

Oversecretion of the adrenal cortex

Due to the close functional connection between the anterior pituitary and the adrenal cortex any excessive secretion of ACTH would result in raised levels of circulating steroids. Oversecretion can be the result of tumours and because the organs are composed of glandular tissue the tumours are adenomata.

Cushing's syndrome

The disease was first described by Harvey Cushing, an American neurosurgeon. This condition, caused by an increase in circulating cortisol, occurs in young adults in a ratio of about four females to every male. Because of the variety of hormones involved the clinical picture can vary but certain characteristics are associated with the patient who has Cushing's syndrome.

Like many endocrine disorders Cushing's syndrome develops over many months or even years. The symptoms have been classically described and a patient developing the disorder will demonstrate some of them. There is moderate or severe obesity of the face and trunk, but not the extremities which become thinner. A pad of fat forms over the dorsal spine which Cushing described as a 'buffalo hump'. The face is moon shaped and the cheeks rosy red. Because of the stretched skin over the abdominal wall and thighs the superficial blood vessels rupture and cause vertical lines called striae. The patient's skin is thin, bruises easily and she tends to suffer from acne of the face. The disturbances of metabolism inhibit the proper healing of cuts or wounds. Hirsutism may be limited to a slight moustache or extend to an abnormal growth of hair over the body – in men there may be a reduction of body hair.

When the patient is admitted to hospital for investigation the main nursing problem is to relieve the patient's embarrassment created by her physical appearance. Privacy and a good relationship is important but this may be hampered by the patient's depressed moods which can vary from self consciousness to severe withdrawal. Mental changes may occur with this disorder and the nurse must not be diverted by the difficulty in communicating with her patient. The nurse should explain any nursing procedures or tests before they begin as this will relieve the patient's apprehension and more co-operation is achieved if she is aware of what is happening.

Diagnostic tests

A test to estimate plasma cortisol will probably show an abnormally high level in Cushing's syndrome. This test can be made using the 'diurnal variation' method. This is based on the fact that plasma cortisol levels vary according to the time of day. A decrease of fifty per cent. normally occurs between early morning readings and those taken at 6 pm but in Cushing's syndrome no change is found.

Examination of urine for 17 – oxogenic steroids is made on a twenty-four hour specimen. This steroid fraction is excreted in large amounts when plasma cortisol is high, the reason for this is not clearly understood. In this test all urine passed during twenty-four hours is collected in a bottle prepared and issued by the laboratory.

Polyuria is often one of the symptoms associated with Cushing's syndrome, it is related to the glycosuria caused by the interference with the action of insulin by cortisol. It is important that nurses maintain accurate recordings of fluid intake and output during investigation. Cortisol also creates a mild degree of hypertension and the physician may order regular estimations of blood pressure as a diagnostic measure.

Various X-rays are taken, including the skull in case of a pituitary tumour; the bones of the spine to eliminate a metabolic disturbance of bone structure; and the chest to show a bronchial tumour which may be associated with this disorder. Each of these X-rays can be considered a diagnostic aid or may detect complications that occur. The patient needs an explanation of what is to take place in the X-ray department. The unknown is frightening to everyone but particularly so for a patient who may be already disturbed by her admission. An X-ray is a painless procedure generally and patients should not be subjected to unnecessary dread before having such a test.

Treatment

The treatment of Cushing's syndrome is dependent upon the cause. The most common reason is enlargement (hyperplasia) of the adrenal cortex through excessive secretion of ACTH from the pituitary gland, which may show a minute adenoma. The adrenal enlargement can be treated by surgical removal of the affected tissue (adrenalectomy). One gland may be removed, or one gland and part of the other (sub-total adrenalectomy), or both glands (total adrenalectomy). There are considerable problems involved in this operation due to the patient's physical condition and her predisposition to wound infection and poor healing.

Nursing care of adrenalectomy

The patient plays a major part in her own recovery, both by cooperating in the treatment given and in being relaxed and as cheerful as possible. Neither of these things can be expected of her however unless she is adequately prepared both physically and mentally. Unless the surgeon has some reason for witholding information the patient should be told what is wrong with her and what the treatment involves. It must be stressed here that the patient should be aware of her treatment before she can sign a consent to operation form and this point needs emphasis as it is sometimes the responsibility of the nursing staff to ensure that the form is completed correctly.

If a good attitude to the treatment is established with the nurse's support the patient will feel less anxious and the result of the operation is more likely to be successful. Routine physical preparation is carried out including a shave from nipple to knee for both sexes – because of the tendency to hirsuitism.

Intramuscular cortisone will be started the day prior to operation when an average dose is 100mg. This is the beginning of replacement therapy to counteract the acute adrenocortical insufficiency which follows the removal of these glands. On returning from theatre the dose of cortisone will be repeated six hourly for twenty-four hours. The post-operative intravenous infusion will also contain steroids, possibly in the form of hydrocortisone. After the critical post-operative phase the dose will be reduced to a maintenance level if total adrenalectomy has been performed. This will continue for the remainder of the patient's life. If a subtotal adrenalectomy is performed then assessment of the patient's remaining hormone secretions will be carried out before more permanent therapy is commenced.

Because of the loss of mineralocorticoids a serious imbalance of body water and salts (electrolytes) will develop. In order to correct this as soon as possible it is essential that nurses check and record accurately the patient's blood pressure and fluid balance. Any deviation from normal should be reported immediately. As the operation is on a site near the diaphragm the patient will be unwilling to breathe deeply because it is painful. To avoid respiratory complications intensive physiotherapy should be started to encourage correct breathing. Nurses should be instructed in these movements to assist the patient during times when the physiotherapist is not in attendance. It is also important to carry out passive exercises on the lower limbs to reduce the risk of deep vein thrombosis.

Surgical removal of an endocrine gland creates a deficiency that will be compensated by drugs and it is vital that nurses follow directions for their administration carefully. Cortisone and any drugs for mineral replacement, including those given by intravenous infusion, must be administered at the times prescribed. Because of poor wound healing and a greater chance of infection in the adrenalectomy patient all sterile procedures must be carried out with meticulous care. Sepsis would complicate the patient's general recovery and cause greater difficulty in hormone balance.

Complications

The major complication of total adrenalectomy is adrenal crisis. This is a condition of collapse caused by changes in fluid balance, electrolytes and circulatory failure. It does not occur immediately following operation but nine to twelve hours later. The patient will complain of greater weakness, anorexia, abdominal pain, severe headache and possibly diarrhoea. On examination the nurse will find her patient's blood pressure extremely low – it may be too low to record. The pulse will be weak and the general picture is of a shocked, anxious patient with a cold, clammy skin.

This is an acute condition and without immediate treatment it would lead to coma followed by death. The sister will report the crisis to the duty surgeon who will order emergency measures, including administration of cortisone by mouth if the patient is not vomiting. An intravenous infusion will probably be needed and the nurse assisting should prepare the equipment in advance. If circulatory failure persists a vasoconstrictor such as noradrenaline will be required. This will be given through the infusion, 5 to 10 micrograms per minute will be sufficient to raise the blood pressure to 100 systolic and maintain it at that level.

Mention should be made here of other conditions that give rise to adrenal crisis.

Addison's disease (see page 97) can produce adrenal crisis, the primary cause varies but the clinical picture remains the same.
Adrenal apoplexy (Waterhouse – Friderichsen syndrome). In this condition the patient has a high temperature and may have a petechial rash with extensive bruising. The cause is a massive septicaemia resulting in necrosis of the adrenal glands. *Adrenal crisis* can result from withdrawal of therapeutic hormones if the patient is reliant upon artificial hormones due to insufficient natural adrenal secretion.

Adrenogenital syndromes

Just as Cushing's syndrome is caused by excessive secretion of glucocorticoids so the adrenogenital syndrome is also caused by one particular steroid group, the androgens.

The androgenic compounds are known as 17 ketosteroids. They are found in the urine, the amount being lower in females because of the masculinising activity. One indicator of adrenogenital disorder is a change in the level of 17 ketosteroids in a twenty-four hour specimen of urine.

The action of androgens is anabolic (building up) and this involves the conversion of amino acids to form tissues continuously throughout life to counteract wear, disease and growth. They become more active at puberty and are concerned directly with the growth of axillary and pubic hair – typical examples of secondary sex development. Secondary characteristics develop in both sexes through the action of androgens together with the hormone produced by the gonads. Thus the action of androgens offset by ovarian hormones are sufficient to induce female development without masculinity. Males develop with the aid of testicular hormones.

Adrenogenital syndromes in children

Androgen disorders may cause malformation before birth. At this stage of growth profound physical change can only be noticed in females. This presents as abnormal development of the external genitalia where it may in extreme cases remain undiagnosed and they may be considered male children. This is due to abnormal development of the clitoris which tends to protrude and can be mistaken for the male penis. These women will eventually have a male build, a deep voice and a male distribution of body hair. Fortunately such extremes are not common.

Male children show no abnormalities at birth but tend to reach puberty at about five years of age when secondary sex characteristics become apparent. Both sexes grow fast because of the anabolic effect of high androgen levels. Growth stops early and the epiphyses in the bones fuse at an earlier age than normal.

Adrenogenital syndromes in adults
As androgens are essentially male hormones the result of oversecretion can only be detected in females. They display typical masculine features such as receding hair and patches of baldness, hair on the face, body and limbs, loss of feminine fat and replacement by masculine muscle. The breasts atrophy and the normal menstrual cycle is disturbed with eventual amenorrhoea, but libido is present because increased androgens increase the heterosexual drive. This picture is that of extreme cases which are not common, the majority demonstrating less pronounced symptoms. Diagnosis is made on the physical signs and confirmed by testing a twenty-four hour specimen of urine which has a raised level of 17 ketosteroids.

Treatment
Treatment is directed at the cause of the condition. If an adenoma is found it will require surgical removal. If the cause of the excessive secretion of androgens is not apparent a synthetic steroid can be given in an effort to reduce the androgen output. Prednisone or dexamethasone can be effective but careful control of the prescribed amounts is necessary.

Conn's syndrome
Conn's syndrome, or primary aldosteronism, is caused by excessive secretion of the mineralocorticoid aldesterone. This is an extremely rare disease unlikely to be seen in the average hospital ward.

The clinical picture reflects a disturbance of electrolytes and water balance. The patient suffers from polyuria and general weakness of the limbs associated with an upset of calcium and potassium levels affecting the function and tone of muscle tissue. Treatment of Conn's syndrome is by removal of the tumour that causes oversecretion.

Undersecretion of the adrenal cortex

Insufficient or complete lack of hormones from the adrenal cortex can result from two distinct causes.

1 Primary failure of the gland to secrete its hormones

2 Secondary failure due to lack of the trophic hormone ACTH from the pituitary gland

Secondary failure is considered in the chapter on the pituitary gland. Primary failure can be attributed to adrenal apoplexy (page 94), acute and chronic infection including tuberculosis and failure for no apparent reason (idiopathic).

Addison's disease

Addison's disease is a condition of cortical atrophy with two main causes. Either primary idiopathic failure or secondary destruction of the gland by tuberculosis, which with the greater therapeutic control of tuberculosis is now rare. The disorder can affect either sex equally and usually appears during the middle years of life. It develops slowly and the symptoms only become noticeable when the patient finds difficulty in managing his normal life without help.

The patient does not complain of any specific illness only a continuous feeling of tiredness which seems to increase as the day passes. He may feed depressed and is prone to minor infections from which he suffers unduly – a simple cold in the head can linger for weeks. A raised level of melanin in the skin causes pigmentation particularly on the nipples and around areas of friction such as the elbows, axillae and the waist where clothes are tight. The patient loses weight in almost every instance and is sometimes dehydrated. Sex characteristics are retained and gonadal function is not affected. The patient comes to hospital to have the diagnosis confirmed.

Unless the possibility of tuberculosis has been eliminated the physician may require isolation until laboratory tests prove negative. Such isolation precautions should be explained to the patient who might otherwise feel he is being isolated because of the appearance of his skin.

Patients with Addison's disease are prone to infection particularly of the respiratory and gastro-intestinal tracts. Efforts are needed to reduce his exposure to infection during the early days of diagnosis and treatment when he is most susceptible. His bed should not be near that of a patient with an infectious disorder, however mild, because of the risk of cross infection. He will have a low blood pressure with a diastolic reading of less than 50mg and a systolic of under 100mg Hg. His blood pressu measurement must be taken and recorded accurately during the initial stages of treatment to allow assessment of his progress to be made. Dizziness can accompany the hypotension and if the patient complains of this the staff should help him when walking to reduce the chance of injury from falling.

Other symptoms such as tachycardia, vomiting and diarrhoea are common and distressing to the patient. Reassurance and an explanation that such problems will disappear as treatment progresses will help the patient to relax. The importance of early recognition of adrenal crisis has been stressed in this chapter. The patient with Addison's disease can suffer a crisis of this type and the nurses must be aware of the signs to summon assistance in an emergency.

Diagnostic tests

Urinalysis

Examination of the patient's urine will show the level of steroids excreted. A low level of aldosterone or the hormone fraction 17 – hydroxycorticoid indicate Addison's disease.

Kepler's water test

This test is extremely efficient in diagnosis of Addison's disease. In preparation the patient must fast from midnight before the test is performed.

a The patient empties his bladder completely before the test starts.
b He is given one litre of water to drink in fifteen minutes if possible.
c He remains in bed for five hours during which time all urine is saved.
d After this time the total is measured, if less than 500ml is passed adrenal insufficiency is probable. Normal subjects pass 700ml or more.

e The test may be repeated after giving the patient cortisone. If he then passes over 700ml the diagnosis is confirmed.

Treatment

The drug of choice is cortisone acetate, 75mg daily in three equally divided doses. The patient will show a marked improvement in one or two weeks, being stronger and less depressed. Deoxycortone acetate may be prescribed if mineralocorticoid replacement is needed. When the patient has returned to a fit condition his drug regime will be reviewed and maintenance doses ordered which he will continue to take for the remainder of his life.

Oversecretion of the adrenal medulla

Functions of the adrenal medulla are related to the autonomic nervous system and the body's reaction to stress. Nervous stimulation causes an outpouring of adrenaline that results in constriction of the peripheral vessels allowing more blood to be available to the muscles. It constricts visceral vessels and dilates the bronchioles, raises the blood pressure and increases cardiac output to prepare the body for 'flight and fight' – a possible survival from the age when man had to protect himself from predatory beasts. This condition of tension is transitory and quickly passes when the primary stimulus disappears.

There is one notable condition that causes an excess of hormones from the adrenal medulla – phaeochromocytoma (phaeos: dusky, chroma: colour, cytos: cell, oma: tumour.) This is a tumour of the dark coloured cells of the medulla as against the light coloured cortical tissue. It is a rare condition usually affecting people of either sex between the ages of twenty and forty-five. The signs and symptoms are merely an exaggeration of the normal function of the hormone. The patient has spasmodic attacks of palpitations, sweating, anxiety and mild trembling of the limbs. Between the attacks he is untroubled by the condition. Treatment is the removal of the offending tumour. This is a most difficult operation because of the fluctuation of blood pressure that occurs when the catecholamine secreting part of the gland is disturbed. During the operation there may be a sudden increase or decrease of catecholamines with a corresponding change in blood pressure. Post-operatively the patient may suffer from permanent hypotension.

Undersecretion of the adrenal medulla

The function of this part of the gland is not essential to life and any deficiency presents no clinical signs of disease. A lack of catecholamines can leave the person with less nervous responses in stress situations which could present problems at times but create no continuous disorder.

General therapeutic use of steroids

Since steroids were first isolated a greater understanding of their function has been possible and the therapeutic use of these drugs has made many advances. Special attention is given to the glucocorticoid group and its physiological effects including the ability to supress the inflammatory process by anti-inflammatory and anti-allergic actions. Cortisol and its analogues can be used to reduce inflammation in a number of disorders unrelated to the endocrine system.

Rheumatism

Steroids are used to relieve joint pains in acute rheumatoid arthritis when they may be taken by mouth or they can be injected directly into the joints.

Status asthmaticus

This disorder responds well to steroid therapy. Once the acute phase is passed the dose is reduced and stopped with no ill effects to the patient.

Inflammation of the gastro-intestinal system

Inflammatory conditions such as ulcerative colitis and regional ileitis can be relieved by steroids in the form of enemata and suppositories.

Ophthalmic conditions

Inflammatory conditions of the eye, particularly in the anterior segment, improve by local application of steroids often combined with antibiotics.

Dermatitis
Skin rashes, particularly those caused by allergic reactions, will improve with direct application of steroids. Certain types of pruritis are also relieved by steroid creams.

Complications
Although therapeutic steroids are invaluable in modern medicine great care is needed in their use. Short term therapy rarely presents serious problems particularly if low doses are used, but continuous use of high doses can cause complications which must be considered before prolonged treatment is commenced.

a Steroids can cause an increase in weight similar to the symptoms of Cushing's syndrome because they cause the patient to retain water in excess of normal.
b The action of the drug can cause sodium retention and a proportional loss of potassium with resulting muscle weakness. Some patients are likely to become hypertensive.
c Because the inflammatory process is reduced prolonged steroid therapy can expose the patient to a recurrence of chronic infections such as tuberculosis. The absence of normal tissue reaction to infection can mask the symptoms and delay treatment.
d Prolonged steroid therapy may accelerate bone changes in the elderly including osteoporosis and subsequent vertebral collapse.
e Patients with latent diabetic symptoms can produce active signs of diabetes mellitus which will require corrective treatment.

If steroids are suddenly withdrawn an adrenal crisis is a serious danger. To prevent this catastrophe the patient should be aware of the importance of taking the drugs regularly as prescribed and warned of the effects if they are stopped without medical supervision.

A patient having steroid therapy should always carry a steroid card giving particulars of his treatment. In an accident or emergency it is essential that the doctor giving treatment should be aware of the steroid treatment and take steps to avoid complications. This is most important when surgical procedures are planned.

Methods of administration of steroids

Steroids are prescribed to be taken orally whenever possible. This is a simple method and once a regular routine is established it is not difficult to take each dose at the correct time. This is an important point with the elderly patient.

Steroids are applied locally in the form of cream or ointment in skin conditions. Fluid suspensions are produced for instillation into the eye or ear. Suppositories and enemata containing steroid drugs are used for direct application to the lower bowel.

A limited number of steroid hormones have been produced in crystal or pellet form for implantation into the superficial muscle tissue for slow, continuous absorption. The sites used include the lower abdominal wall and the thigh, using local anaesthetic and strict aseptic conditions. Replacement is necessary after six to eight months.

6
Sexual Development

Members of the human race are divided into two distinct types, male and female and throughout their existence this primary division plays a major part. The division of the sexes is responsible for separate mental attitudes and physical variations, different modes of growth and structure and different functions in life. Sex is determined at the moment of fertilisation, when the gametes (sperm and ovum) unite. The body contains two types of cells, the somatic cells which form tissues and organs and the reproductive cells necessary for continuance of the species. The number of cells are constantly changing as some die and are replaced. The new cells are created by binary fission, a process in which each cell divides into two by splitting. Somatic cells divide by mitosis giving body cells for replacement and growth, each an exact replica of the original. Reproductive gametes divide by the process of meiosis. These cells are similar except for an important difference in the number of chromosomes in the nucleus.

Chromosomes are minute structures in the nucleus of each cell which are essential for organised growth. Without the chromosomal 'key' to guide it the growth process would be an uncontrolled action only allowing a similar specimen to develop through remote chance. Chromosomes are the plans of the future organism whose size, colour and other characteristics they determine. Here we are concerned with the effects of the endocrine system on sexual development.

Within the nucleus of each somatic cell there are forty-six chromosomes, formed into twenty-three pairs of which twenty-two pairs are related to body growth and called autosomes; the remaining pair is related to sex development and are called sex chromosomes. The sex chromosomes are called X and Y, in females the pair consist of X and X, in males they are X and Y. In reproductive cell division the twenty-two pairs of autosomes are divided and one chromosome of each pair goes into each new cell that develops from the fission. The sex chromosomes also divide one to each cell. The results of this division are two reproductive cells, each female ovum contains twenty-two autosomes and one X sex chromo-

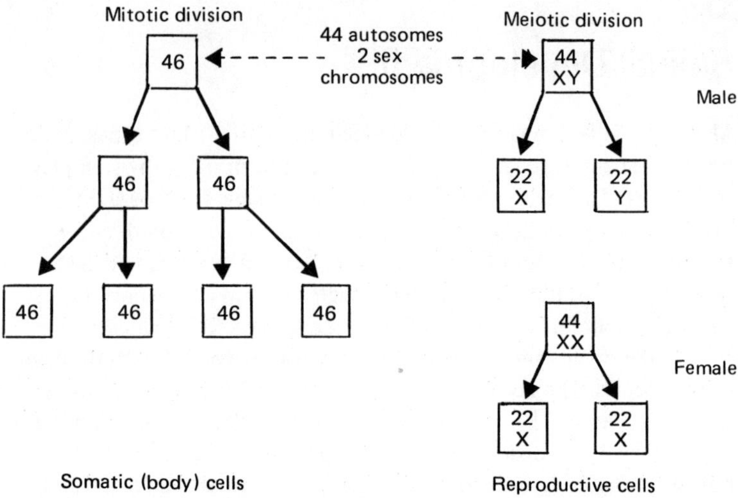

Fig 6:1 Cell division

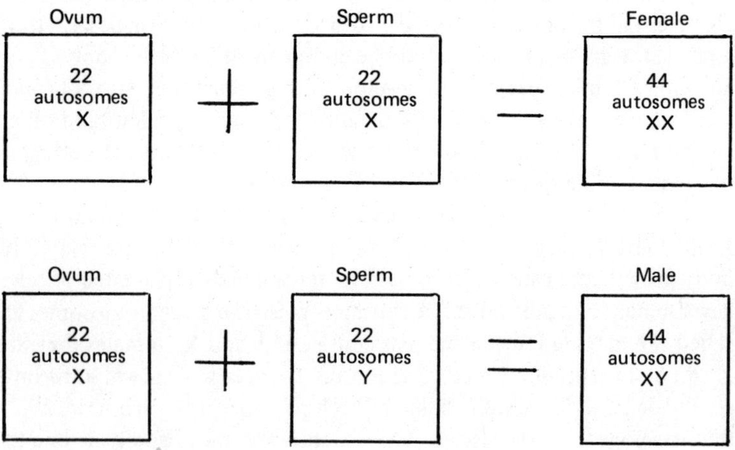

Fig 6:2 Determination of sex

some whilst each male sperm contains twenty-two autosomes and either one X or one Y sex chromosome.

When fertilisation occurs one sperm unites with one ovum and in doing so creates a new chromosomal pattern. The combination results in twenty-two pairs of autosomes and one pair of sex chromosomes – it is at this point that the sex of the embryo is decided. Each female reproductive cell can contribute one X chromosome to the union, while the male cell contains either one X or one Y. There is an equal chance of either one being involved in the combination. If the sperm provides an X the resulting pair X X will develop into a female, if alternatively a Y is used the pair X Y will develop into a male.

This random chance is necessary for the numbers of males and females to be nearly equal at any one time. Because of a similarity in the composition of either sex the primary development of the reproductive system is from an anatomical source able to grow into either tract. In early embryonic life primitive gonads form on the posterior wall of the abdominal cavity as a structure which consists of two distinct systems known as the Wolffian and Mullerian ducts. At about the twelfth week of foetal life one of them develops while the other degenerates and disappears. If the Wolffian duct remains it becomes the male reproductive system and if the Mullerian duct continues to grow it develops into the female reproductive system. Although the unrequired system degenerates, the fact that some vestiges of its tissue remain can be demonstrated by minute amounts of circulating hormone not related to the dominant tract. It is thought they play a part in the delicate balance of hormone levels during the years of childhood when growth and development is at a maximum, and on into adult life.

Puberty

During the early years of childhood growth continues without any great influence being brought to bear by the gonads. Their action, in conjunction with gonadtrophins and the adrenal cortex, become more evident at the age of puberty. It is at this time that secondary sex characteristics are noticeable and changes occur which are influenced by this complex hormonal pattern. In males the signs of puberty are derived from the adrenal glands and the testis, under the influence of pituitary trophic hormones. Changes include growth of axillary and body hair, enlargement of the external genitalia and deepening of the voice. In contrast to the new growth of hair on the body there may be a recession of the hair line on the head which continues during adult life. In females the changing pattern is stimulated by a rise of oestrogen levels which causes growth of pubic and axillary hair, rounding of body contours and the development of breast tissue. In the reproductive tract there is an enlargement of the uterus and the beginning of endometrial growth, in preparation for the onset of the menstrual cycle (menarche).

The changes of puberty occur at about thirteen years in girls and a little later in boys. The whole process of puberty is slow and although it falls between the ages of twelve to fifteen physical maturation continues until adulthood.

Menopause

The menopause occurs naturally in both sexes, in women it takes place between the ages of forty and fifty whilst in men the equivalent testicular failure may not become evident until over sixty years. The change in women, which is much more noticeable, is attributed to failure of the ovary to respond to stimulation of trophic hormones, possibly due to exhaustion of viable Graffian follicles. The disparity in the menopausal ages of different women may be due to some variation in the number of functional follicles. Masculine failure has no comparable problem as spermatozoa are not secreted from such a limited source. Menopausal symptoms may be induced by surgical removal of testes or ovaries, in which case the signs will be more dramatic than when following the normal pattern.

When the hormonal secretion ceases the organs of the system show changes. The uterus shrinks, the cervix atrophies and the external genitalia atrophy and stop secreting, body hair is lost and breasts lose their shape. These physical changes are accompanied by physiological and psychological differences that are the outward signs of the menopause. There is a change in the menstrual cycle when the intervals between each period become longer or the flow can appear scanty and stop. Disturbances in the circulatory system cause palpitations and dizziness, and transient hypertension gives characteristic 'hot flushes'. The woman complains of feeling constantly tired and unable to concentrate. She may be depressed for no apparent reason; headaches and joint pains can occur.

Most women can adjust to this normal pattern of change without undue difficulty. In order to adapt successfully a woman needs to develop new attitudes to her function in life. The fact that she has passed the reproductive and child bearing age need not diminish her sense of fulfilment any more than it should upset her sexual activity. She will find it easier to forget about the changes taking place if she concerns herself with new interests and hobbies as much as possible. Occasionally exaggerated symptoms may demand hormonal assistance during this time. If it is thought advisable to supplement the patient's hormone pattern in an effort to minimise the symptoms synthetic hormones may be prescribed. Stilboestrol can be used in small doses.

Disorders of sexual development

Disorders connected with abnormal maturation can develop during the early years of growth though some may not become apparent until puberty when dysfunction is noticed.

Precocious puberty

Precocious puberty means development of the signs of puberty at an early age, indeed instances are recorded as early as three to four years of age.

Male precocity

Early stimulation of the adrenal cortex from the pituitary, tumours of the adrenal cortex or a tumour of the interstitial cells of the testis can produce this condition. Development can follow a pattern consistent with normal puberty and treatment is directed at the primary cause of the condition. Surgery is sometimes necessary, particularly if tumours are responsible.

Female precocity
A similar condition arising in girls causes premature menstrual bleeding and breast growth. Causes include ovarian tumours. Again treatment is directed at the cause of the accelerated changes.

Delayed puberty
Certain conditions may retard puberty for several years, even to the age of twenty, whilst others cause permanent loss of sex development for life. Some may develop late from an unknown cause giving no permanent ill effects. In other more serious cases, puberty is never reached due to gonadal failure or ineffective pituitary stimulation.

Genetic disorders
The means by which the chromosome content of each body cell consists of forty-four autosomes and two sex chromosomes has been briefly described already. It will be appreciated that faulty division of a reproductive cell could vary the distribution of sex chromosomes. If the sex chromosomes do not separate into their respective gametes at the time of the cell division the result will be one cell with two sex chromosomes and one containing none. When conjugation occurs the total chromosomal count will not be true. There are many variations of the chromosome number possible but only two are mentioned here.

1 A chromosome count of forty-seven, showing the addition of one extra sex chromosome ie XXY (Klinefelter's syndrome) – males.
2 A chromosome count of forty-five, indicating a deficiency of one sex chromosome ie XO (Turner's syndrome) – females.

Klinefelter's syndrome
This is characterised by a lack of secondary sex development, with small testes and often some breast growth; these men tend to be tall with extra growth in the legs. The condition may not be discovered until puberty or when infertility or loss of libido is found. It is related to lack of development of the interstitial cells of the testis. Klinefelter's syndrome is often associated with low intelligence, but this is not always so and the patient can have a normal intelligence level. Treatment of

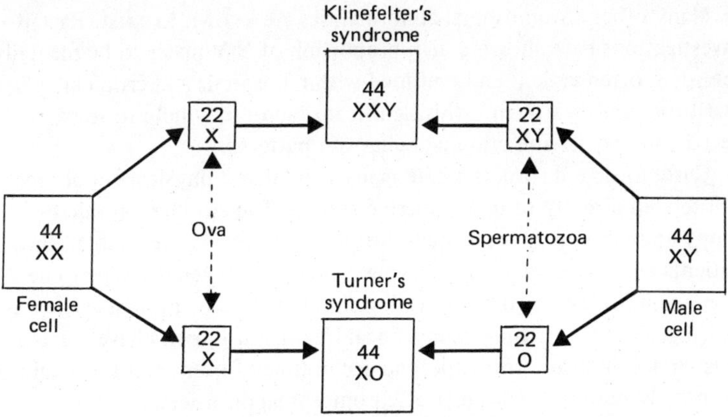

Fig 6:3 Chromosomal abnormalities

this condition is of little value as there is a minimal chance of inducing spermatogenesis and potency due to malformation of the testes.

Turner's syndrome

This condition may be noticed before puberty because of the appearance of specific physical signs. There is often a web-like skin fold growing from each side of the neck, breast development is absent and the body contours are masculine with wide shoulders and narrow hips. The patient is usually short in stature and lacking in pubic and axillary hair. A condition of increased angling at the elbow joint, known as cubitus valgus, is present. Although the uterus and vagina are intact there is complete amenorrhoea, the ovaries being only vestiges of inactive tissue. There may be pigmentation over the neck and chest. Treatment of this condition is difficult but, if diagnosed early, hormone therapy may induce some cyclical bleeding. This can be of psychological benefit, although the patient will be infertile due to a lack of natural ovarian hormones. In younger patients oestrogen can increase the chance of breast development giving the patient a greater sense of femininity.

Many other chromosomal abnormalities are known to exist. Recent investigations have shown a high proportion of Y Y males to be mentally retarded, often violent and confined within hospitals and criminal institutions. Research into this significant factor may help to solve certain anti-social and criminal behaviour patterns.

Chromosome disorders create many mental and physical conditions not related directly to the endocrine system. The advances in microscopy and laboratory techniques during recent years have enabled those patients who are suspected of having problems of a genetic type to be advised about the question of having children. This form of assistance is called genetic counselling. Many Local Health Authorities have created this service and can offer expert advice in time of need, and this could eventually reduce the number of chromosomal disorders.

7

The Testis

The testes are the major secreting organs of the male reproductive system. They consist of two oval shaped structures approximately 5cm long and 3cm wide lying in the scrotum, suspended from the spermatic cord to form part of the external genitalia. They are highly vascular and receive a blood supply from the testicular arteries passing down the abdominal wall and forming part of the spermatic cord. The blood

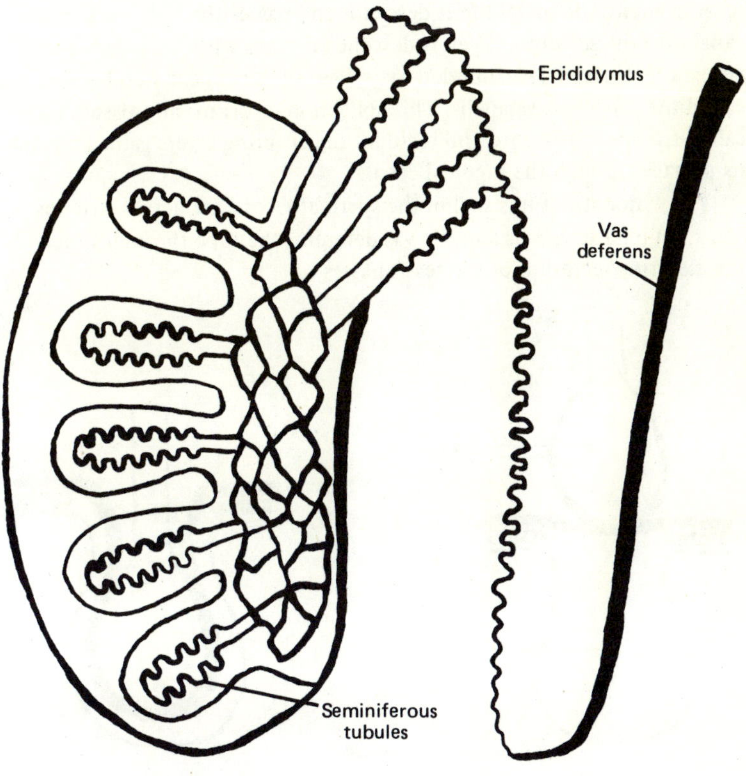

Fig 7:1 Structure of the testis

returns through the testicular veins following a similar course. The nerve supply originates from the thoracic nerves, their function is to constrict and dilate the blood vessels within the glands.

The outer surface of the testis is covered by a thin membrane, the tunica vaginalis, which originates from the peritoneum. Under this membrane is attached a thicker coat, the tunica albuginae. Radiating from the posterior aspect of the testis are many tortuous tubes called the seminiferous tubules, they form a large part of the testis and meet to form a collecting tubule called the epididymis.

The testis develops on the posterior abdominal wall. At about the seventh month of foetal life it descends and passes through the inguinal canal into the scrotum. When it descends it takes with it a number of necessary structures surrounded by a sheet of peritoneal membrane called the processus vaginalis. This collection of organs and tissues is called the spermatic cord and includes the covering layers gained during its passage through the inguinal canal.

The major structures within the spermatic cord are nerves, arteries, veins, lymphatic vessels and the vas deferens, the tube through which the exocrine secretion of the testis passes.

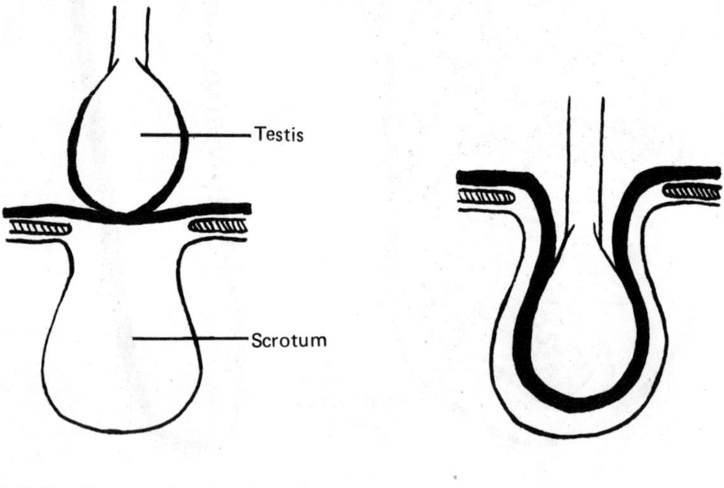

Fig 7:2 Descent of the testis into the scrotum

Between the seminiferous tubules are clusters of cells called Leydig's cells which secrete the hormones of the testis. The seminiferous tubules are lined with groups of large swollen cells responsible for reproduction and the production of gametes or spermatozoa. Spermatogenesis (the action of producing spermatozoa) starts about the time of puberty and continues throughout life. There is normally no change in cell structure during the later years but some inconsistency of function is usual.

The endocrine function of the testis arises from the cells of Leydig. The principal hormone is testosterone which is sometimes referred to as an androgen because of its similar action to the hormone secreted by the adrenal cortex. The development of the testis is controlled by two pituitary gonadotrophins which are secreted in minimal amounts before puberty when testicular growth is slow. At puberty Interstitial Cell Stimulating Hormone (ICSH) stimulates interstitial cells to secrete testosterone and Follicle Stimulating Hormone (FSH) activates the seminiferous tubules to produce gametes.

The pituitary gonadotrophins are essential for the production of testosterone and failure of the anterior pituitary gland will cause the testes to atrophy. If both testes fail to function from some other cause resulting in a reduction of circulating testosterone the gonadotrophin level will rise in an effort to stimulate the organs to secrete. This only occurs if both testes fail to function as one active testis secretes sufficient hormone to control pituitary stimulation. There is also an intricate relationship between testosterone and adrenal androgens which is important in the development of secondary sex characteristics. Endocrine disorders of the testis can be divided into hyposecretion and hypersecretion.

Hyposecretion

Hyposecretion, or hypogonadism, can result in two separate deficiencies because of the double function in secreting testosterone and spermatozoa. The causes of failure to secrete testosterone are divided into two groups.

1 Primary, caused by a disorder of the testis.
2 Secondary, from a failure of the pituitary trophic hormone.

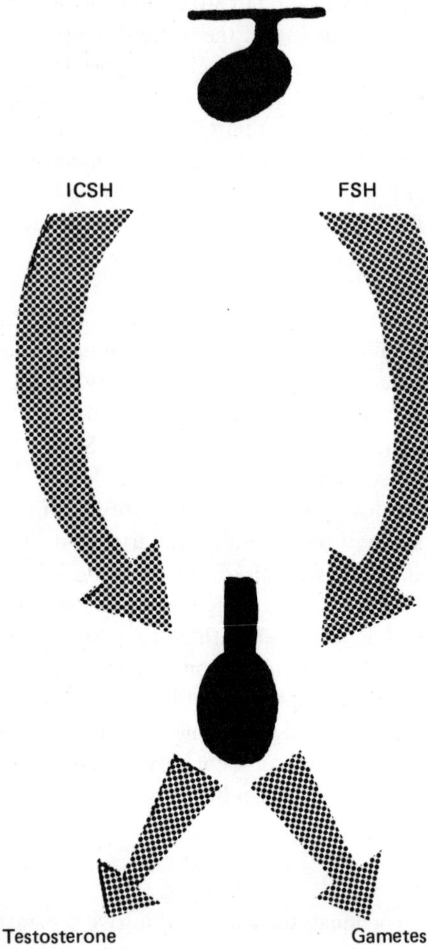

Fig 7:3 Pituitary control of the testis

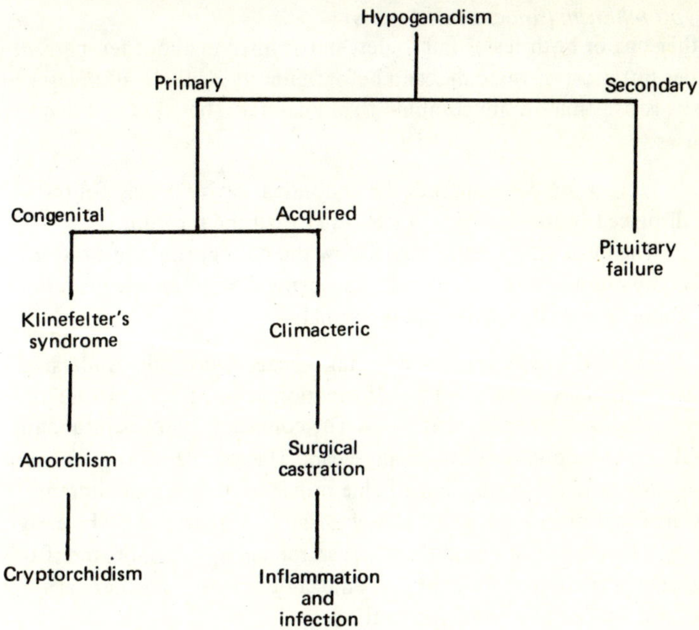

Fig 7:4 Causes of hypogonadism

Primary hypogonadism

Congenital

Klinefelter's syndrome
This is a condition resulting from a chromosomal disorder. It is discussed in the chapter on sexual development (page 108).

Anorchism
This is a congenital defect in which the testes fail to develop and often only vestiges of testicular tissue are present. It is a rare condition and results in loss of all testicular function.

Cryptorchidism (undescended testis)
Either one or both testes fail to descend at birth in about ten percent of males but most of these descend before puberty. Unilateral undescended testis is five times more common than bilateral. There are two main causes.

1 During the descent from the abdominal cavity it may follow a displaced route leading to a site other than the scrotum.
2 The descending testis may follow the correct route but fail to complete its descent and remain suspended between the posterior abdominal wall and the inguinal canal.

The reason why cryptorchidism takes place is not fully understood but it is thought to be due to malformation or insufficient stimulus from the gonadotrophic hormones. The condition is not painful and could remain undetected for many years. The excellent programme of diagnostic and preventative medicine provided for school children ensures that most cases of cryptorchidism are discovered in the early years. The chance of a functional organ remaining are improved if this disorder is treated when young. As the child grows older there is a reduced chance of normal maturation.

The best time to start treatment is thought to be between the ages of five and nine years. The treatment depends on the cause, hormonal therapy is used if normal descent is arrested but if the testis is displaced (ectopic testis) the patient will be admitted to hospital for surgery.

As one would expect the child appears healthy and fit on arrival in the ward and he will not complain of any pain or discomfort although he might show a certain amount of apprehension on admission. If he knows the reason for his admission he may well feel embarrassed. As with any other patient the nurse must inspire this young boy's confidence and cooperation and help him to adjust to his new environment by introducing him to the other patients in the ward. She can also allay his anxiety by answering his questions in a sensible manner. It is useless to tell him that it will not hurt when this is not true. When giving the child an injection, for example, she should tell him what she is doing and that it may hurt slightly. He may feel apprehensive at first but will soon realise that he can trust the nurse and when he is told something it is true. Most children prefer to be treated in a grown up manner and will cooperate with their treatment more willingly if they know staff are not trying to deceive them or pretend.

The surgical treatment for cryptorchidism involves freeing the testis and drawing it down into the scrotum, this operation is called orchidopexy. Problems arise when the vessels and nerves attached to the testis are found to be too short and the testis may be removed to prevent complications. When the testis is drawn into the scrotum it requires an attachment to retain it in position for the first few weeks. The scrotum is opened and the testis sutured to the fascia of the thigh. After six to eight weeks the sutures are removed and the scrotum incision closed. The testis can also be retained by passing a suture through the strong covering of the tunica albuginae and attaching it to the scrotal wall.

Orchidectomy is only performed when absolutely necessary, in particular if both testes are involved. Complete castration (bilateral orchidectomy) causes loss of all hormonal and reproductive function, it is the practice therefore to leave one functional testis when possible. If an undescended testis cannot be brought down it is best removed as complications develop if left in the abdominal cavity. There is complete loss of spermatogenesis while the testis is in the abdominal cavity due to the constant body heat. In the scrotum the testis, by muscular contraction, is able to move toward or away from the body according to its environmental temperature. The exposure to a constant heat of 37°C stops the activity of the seminiferous tubules. The possibility of torsion is greater if the testis is in an incorrect position and this could require surgical treatment. The most important reason for removal of an undescended testis is the high risk of malignancy during the early years of adult life and as it does not function nothing is gained by allowing it to remain.

If arrested descent is the cause of cryptorchidism hormone therapy may be attempted before surgery. This is not a very satisfactory method however and the results are often disappointing. The hormone of choice is human chorionic gonadotrophin which may induce the testis to descend spontaneously and without mechanical assistance. When used for disorders of the testis the hormone is given as an intramuscular injection of 500–1,000 units twice weekly for up to eight weeks. If there is no improvement other methods of treatment are considered.

Acquired

Male climateric

There is no specific change in which male reproductive function ceases in a comparable way to the female menopause. Loss of libido and failure to secrete spermatozoa is a gradual process and the body adapts with few effects.

Surgical castration

Removal of both testes will cause immediate hypogonadism and cessation of all secretions with loss of libido.

Inflammation and infection

The testis like other organs and tissues is susceptible to infection. Inflammation of the testis (orchitis) may be caused by syphilis, tuberculosis or more commonly as a complication of an infectious fever, particularly mumps.

Mumps, also called epidemic parotitis, is a virus disease frequently seen in boys between the ages of five and fifteen years. It begins with acute fever accompanied by swelling of the parotid glands in the neck. Orchitis is one of the serious and painful complications that can develop.

During the acute phase the patient will be nursed in bed and complaints of painful testes will indicate orchitis. This is usually confined to boys at or over the age of puberty. About one patient in five suffers with orchitis. The reason is unknown although some organisms have an affinity for certain body tissues and the virus of mumps is thought to be one of these. The testes must be carefully supported and protected as the whole scrotum is extremely painful. It is necessary to take the weight of the bedclothes from the lower abdomen with a bedcradle. The testes can be supported by lengths of Elastoplast stretched across the upper thighs with wrappings of cotton wool for protection and warmth.

It is important to realise the embarrassment a patient of this age will have during treatment and therefore when possible such procedures should be carried out by a male nurse.

Secondary hypogonadism

This is found in males with complete failure of the anterior lobe of the pituitary gland, it is discussed in greater detail in the chapter on pituitary disorders (page 11).

Hypersecretion

Hypersecretion, or hypergonadism, generally arises from two causes, tumours of the adrenal cortex or tumour of the testis. Other causes are rare and of academic interest.

The problem of hypergonadism is a tendency to grow and mature physically at an early age. When it involves boys between the ages of five to fifteen years this abnormal development is called precocious puberty. As the patient grows rapidly so axillary and pubic hair appear and the external genitalia reach adult proportions. In appearance the patient looks much older than his age being both taller and of good muscular development. This advanced development is related to the disturbance of hormone secretion. The relationship between androgens and testosterone in the average maturing male is extremely complex. Although minor variations are not critical a constant change does affect development.

Tumours of the adrenal gland are the common cause and are considered in the chapter on the adrenal gland. Tumours of the testis are uncommon and fall into three main groups.

1 A seminoma which is a malignant tumour affecting the seminiferous tubules. It is the largest group.
2 A teratoma which is a type of tumour composed of tissues foreign to the organ on which it grows.
3 Interstitial cell tumours are extremely rare but affect the tissue concerned with the secretion of sex hormones and can cause precocious puberty.

Treatment for tumours of the testis can be surgery, radiotherapy or a combination of the two. Great care is necessary as there is a high risk of malignancy and metastases can spread easily to adjacent tissues including the complex lymphatic vessels of the pelvis.

Anabolic agents

The action of proteins in the body can be anabolic or catabolic. These changes are continually taking place and form a part of the normal metabolic process. Some conditions create a need for artificial synthesis of proteins in excess of the average requirement and the use of androgens and testosterone is sometimes effective.

Anabolic agents may be used in diseases where loss of weight is evident including conditions causing poor appetite such as congestive cardiac failure, gastro-intestinal diseases, osteoporosis and a number of chronic conditions which keep the patient immobile for long periods. Examples of anabolic agents are Norethandrolone and Nandrolone. Disturbances of diet coupled with diseases causing excessive loss of protein require the patient to replace the body tissue to allow recovery to take place. Outside the field of medicine anabolic agents are used in today's highly competitive realm of sport. Field events demand muscular strength coupled with agility and balance. Competitors can gain an advantage by using such agents in combination with high protein diets.

Prostate gland

Other parts of the male reproductive system that are dependent on hormonal secretions for development include the prostate gland. This is a glandular structure at the base of the bladder surrounding the urethra it secretes prostatic fluid which plays a part in ejaculation. This gland is important, medically, as it has a tendency to enlarge in men after the age of sixty years. The enlargement causes inefficiency of micturition first and later retention as an immediate problem. If untreated there is a greater risk of malignancy. In cancer of the prostate gland the malignant cells need normal hormone levels to remain active. If this balance of hormones is disturbed the growth may be inhibited. Prostatic carcinoma can be treated either by surgery or by hormone therapy. Circulating hormones are changed by castration or by continuous hormone therapy with oestrogen. Stilboestrol is the drug of choice for this condition it is given in doses of 25 mg three times daily. The effect of such measures is to depress the pituitary gland and stop the secretion of trophic hormones to the testis. This can cause side effects such as atrophy of the testes for which the patient should be prepared but as he is likely to be past the age of reproduction this should present few problems. One noticeable complication is the effect of oestrogen on male breast tissue which can grow (gynaecomastia) with mild inflammation. This is reduced by decreasing the dose of oestrogen to a maintenance level after the initial period of treatment.

8
The Ovary

The ovary forms part of the female reproductive system. Patients with disorders of this system are nursed in gynaecological wards. Nurses experienced in this work will be aware that such wards have a special atmosphere of their own. All the patients have diseases of the reproductive system and because of the interdependence of reproduction and the complete female role their problems tend to be emotional as well as physical. Gynaecological patients require both physical and psychological care to help them develop the attitudes needed for a satisfactory recovery. Although this is especially important for those having radical treatment it applies to all patients however minor their problem. Nurses must remember that the patient is suffering from a disorder affecting their natural femininity and they need to be treated with the greatest care and understanding.

The ovaries are two almond shaped organs measuring 3 to 5cm in length. They are situated on each side of the pelvis attached to the posterior aspect of the broad ligament. The broad ligament is a part of the peritoneum which is reflected to support the uterus and fix the ovaries and Fallopian tubes in their natural position. The ovary is also retained in position by the ovarian ligament, a short fibrous cord within the broad ligament. It is essential that the ovary is anatomically secure in its position at the end of the Fallopian, or uterine, tube to allow the ovum to pass into the tube and uterus. The end of the Fallopian tube is near but not attached to the ovary.

They receive a rich blood supply from the ovarian arteries which originate from the abdominal aorta. The ovarian artery joins the uterine artery to form a complex of vessels near the uterine tube. The venous system follows a similar pattern returning blood from the left ovary into the renal vein and from the right ovary into the inferior vena cava. The lymphatic vessels accompany the arteries and veins through the pelvis ending in the aortic lymph glands. Sympathetic and parasympathetic nerves pass down to form a complex around the ovary and control the size of blood vessels serving the organ.

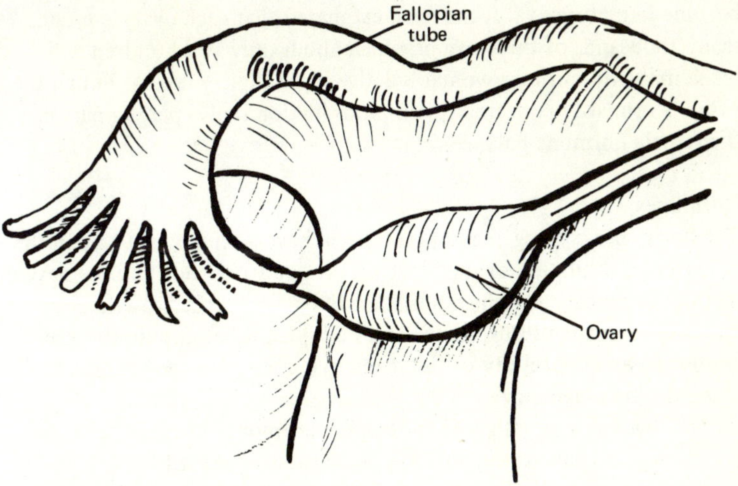

Fig 8:1 Position of ovary and Fallopian tube

The ovaries form an integral part of the reproductive system and their function is related to other structures, the most important of which are the Fallopian tubes and the uterus.

The Fallopian tubes link the ovary and the uterus. Each tube is about 10cm long containing one open end adjacent to the ovary while the other is attached to the uterus. The tubes lie in the upper margins of the broad ligament and are completely covered by the broad ligament except at the dorsal aspect which opens into the pelvic cavity close to the ovary. At the ovarian end of the tube is a mass of minute processes called fimbriae which assist the discharged ovum into the tube.

The secretions of the ovary perform two separate functions.

1 Reproductive cells (ova)
2 Hormones (a. oestrogen, b. progestagen)

Reproductive cells

During early foetal life the ovary develops a large number of undifferentiated cells called primordial cells, or follicles, which eventually become immature ova. It has been estimated that each ovary contains many thousands of these ova of which about only two hundred will reach maturity during a woman's active reproductive life. Although the ovum is primarily concerned with reproduction it also plays a part in the female hormone balance.

Hormones

The hormones oestrogen and progestagen have an important role in the growth and regulation of the female reproductive system and the development of secondary sex characteristics. In particular the growth and maturation of the uterus, vagina and Fallopian tubes at puberty, the regulation and continuity of the menstrual cycle, and the changes that occur during pregnancy.

The ovary is a target gland for trophic hormones of the anterior pituitary gland called gonadotrophins. Without stimulation of these trophic hormones, Follicle Stimulating Hormone and Luteinising Hormone (FSH and LH) the ovary will not function, for example following hypophysectomy. The pituitary gland influences the secretions of the ovary through a regular sequence of gonadotrophins in the non-pregnant female. In pregnancy controlled changes preserve the embryo in the uterus. Stimulation of the ovary is governed by the 'feed back' mechanism where circulating levels of oestrogen and progestagen affect the pituitary gland.

The gonadotrophic hormones:

Follicle stimulating hormone

As its name suggests FSH is related to stimulation of ovarian follicles. Towards the end of each unfertilised menstrual cycle FSH stimulates a follicle to mature and become a Graafian follicle containing a ripe ovum. The Graafian follicle eventually ruptures to release the ovum, a process called ovulation which forms part of the menstrual cycle called the proliferative phase. During this time the ovary secretes oestrogen.

Luteinising hormone

After ovulation the level of FSH diminishes and the pituitary gland secretes LH causing the ruptured follicle to regenerate and form the corpus luteum. The corpus luteum degenerates if fertilisation does not take place leaving a scar of fibrous tissue. This is called the secretory or progestational phase and is followed by the menstrual phase.

Ovarian hormones

Oestrogen

Oestrogen is the collective name for the ovarian steroid group of hormones the most important of which is oestradiol. It is necessary for the development of sex characteristics and the menarche. It is also thought to act on the mucous membrane of the vagina to increase the number of commensal organisms ie Doderlein's bacillus to create an acid environment and give some protection against pathogenic organisms.

Progestagen

The principal hormone in the progestagen group is progesterone, this is secreted by the corpus luteum together with oestrogen. Its physiological action is not completely understood although it is known to affect the lining of the uterus, the endometrium, during the latter half of the menstrual cycle and is associated with breast changes during lactation.

The menstrual cycle

Menstruation is a normal function that becomes an accepted part of female life after puberty. It is important that a child learns to regard menstruation as a normal function in which her health does not suffer. The importance of hygiene should be emphasised. The problem of associated pain can be relieved by mild analgesics such as paracetamol. Menarche usually begins between the ages of twelve and sixteen years and continues until the menopause or during pregnancy. The complete cycle is about twenty-eight days but can vary from three to five weeks and once established it should follow a regular rhythm in each individual.

Although the menstrual cycle is usually considered to begin with the menstrual phase it is easier, with regard to hormone involvement, to start with the proliferative phase. FSH stimulates the development of an ovarian follicle which matures into a Graafian follicle. The ovary secretes oestradiol to encourage the endometrium of the uterus to proliferate

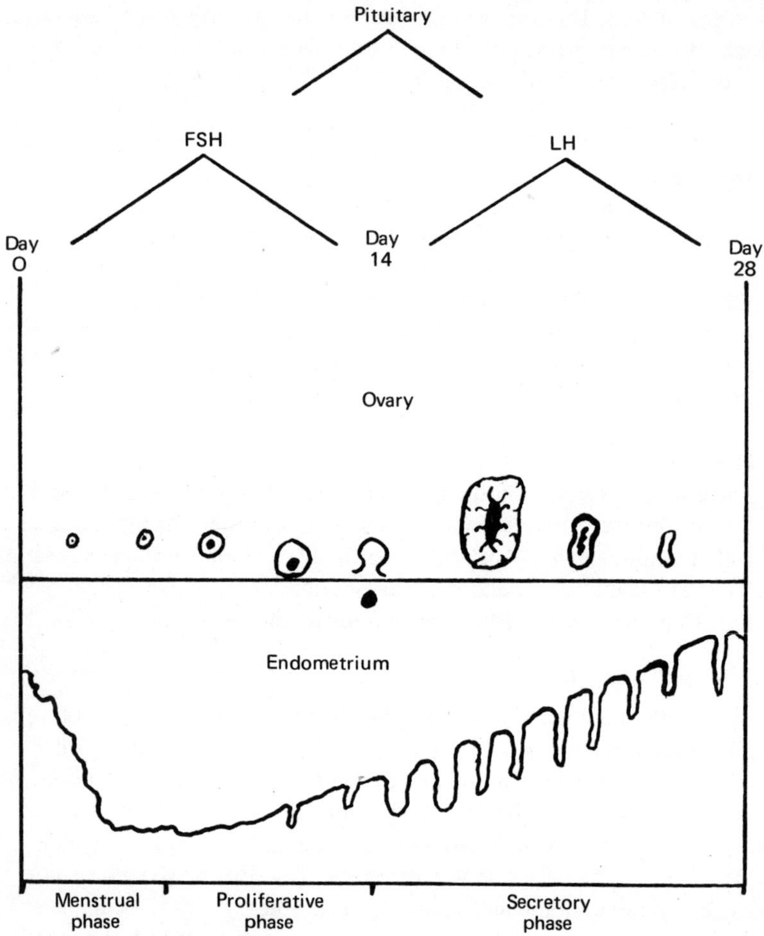

Fig 8:2 The menstrual cycle

and grow – hence the name of this phase of the cycle. Glands and epithelial cells are regenerated and the mass of small blood vessels reform being aided by the high vascularity of the organ. For about ten days the uterus prepares to receive a fertilised ovum and at the end of this time the Graafian follicle ruptures to release the ovum. If fertilisation is to take place it occurs during the movement of the ovum down the Fallopian tube towards the body of the uterus. Spermatozoa penetrate the ovum, fertilisation occurs and cell division begins before implantation into the wall of the uterus. At the time of ovulation the level of FSH diminishes and remains low for the remaining part of the cycle while the level of LH rises. This causes the ovary to secrete progesterone and oestradiol from the corpus luteum. This is the secretory phase of the cycle during which the endometrium becomes thicker and arterioles form in the wall of the uterus. The endometrium secretes glycogen – hence the name of this phase. This continues until five to six days before menstruation is due. If fertilisation does not occur there is a sudden drop in the level of both hormones causing the endometrium to shrink. Secretions of glycogen cease and the minute blood vessels of the uterus go into spasm cutting off the blood supply to the endometrium and the superficial lining falls away. This is the menstrual phase which continues for four to five days after which the process begins again.

Hormone variations in pregnancy

A distinct change occurs in hormone levels when an ovum is fertilised. The corpus luteum continues to enlarge and for several weeks the level of progesterone is increased. This is necessary whilst the embryo develops during the early stages of growth before the placenta is established when this is able to secrete its own hormones during the remainder of the pregnancy. The placental hormone is known as chorionic gonadotrophin and is produced by the chorionic villi of the placenta. Its function is to maintain a high level of progesterone and inhibit the level of FSH in order to prevent the menstrual phase occuring.

Disorders of the ovary

Disorders of the ovary involving hormones may be considered as three groups.

1 Amenorrhoea
2 Dysfunctional uterine bleeding
3 Neoplasms and cysts

Amenorrhoea

The word amenorrhoea means absence of menstruation and is often divided into primary and secondary groups although this may be considered to be an arbitrary classification. Whatever its cause may be, amenorrhoea is due to a non-functioning ovary.

Primary amenorrhoea is the term used to describe a condition in which menstruation has never taken place. It is applied to a female who fails to menstruate at the age of puberty or after. Once common cause of primary amenorrhoea is failure of other endocrine organs. Pituitary defects and cretinism are examples of this, in each of which there is a failure of the ovary through lack of trophic hormone stimulation. Other causes include genetic defects when the reproductive tract has failed to develop completely or organs of the system are absent. Chromosomal defects can be the cause as in Turner's syndrome where there is an almost total absence of ovarian tissue.

A patient with secondary amenorrhoea has menstruated in the past but has not followed a normal cycle for at least two to three months. The common causes are pregnancy and the menopause, the latter being the natural process of ovarian failure in women who have passed the child bearing age. There are endocrine disorders which result in the absence of menstruation, as in the failure of gonadotrophic hormones in Simmond's disease. Untreated myxoedema can lead to amenorrhoea for the same reason. Psychogenic factors also cause amenorrhoea, particularly in young girls who are fearful of becoming pregnant or whilst in times of stress such as during examinations for example. Disorders of the hypothalamus, an important part of the nervous and endocrine systems, can produce the same result. Anorexia nervosa, a condition of hypothalamic origin in which there is a complete loss of appetite, can include amenorrhoea. Secondary amenorrhoea occurs after surgical removal of both ovaries (bilateral oophorectomy) and following excessive irradiation.

Most cases of amenorrhoea are treated medically. One exception is a condition called Stein Leventhal's syndrome where the ovaries become enlarged and multiple cysts develop below the outer capsule of the organ (polycystic disease of the ovary). The patient may complain of secondary amenorrhoea, infertility, obesity and an abnormal growth of hair (hirsutism) over the face and body. Diagnosis is often difficult as the hormones are not completely absent and the administration of progesterone often produces bleeding. Although the cause is unknown it is treated by wedge resection of the ovaries. An operation in which part of the ovary is removed, in most cases it leads to normal cyclical bleeding starting again.

Medical treatment of amenorrhoea

Patients with amenorrhoea may be admitted to hospital for investigations and it is important that a good nurse-patient relationship is established. The patient will be under a severe degree of stress due to her disorder and the anxiety of admission to hospital can cause further emotional problems.

Investigations are limited and not always satisfactory. Assessment of hormones in a series of twenty-four hour urine specimens and a sequence of morning temperature recordings can indicate ovarian activity and the difference in hormone levels compared with a normal cycle. Examination of the vaginal epithelium can show changes as it is affected by hormones in a similar manner to the uterine epithelium. It must be appreciated that amenorrhoea is not a disease but the symptom of a disorder involving an organ of the reproductive system.

If primary amenorrhoea is diagnosed the aim of treatment is to establish a cycle of bleeding by stimulating the ovaries. Oestrogen can be given in order to stimulate a secretory phase in the uterus. It is given in the form of stilboestrol for fourteen days and then stopped, after which bleeding should commence. This is called 'withdrawal bleeding'. If it is not successful the dose may be increased. If regular bleeding is started treatment may be discontinued in some cases as the initial stimulation is all that is required. The administration of oestrogens will also stimulate the development of secondary sex characteristics, breasts, axillary and pubic hair if puberty is retarded. Such changes give the patient a degree of psychological satisfaction and this could be a contributing factor in the development of a regular menstrual cycle.

In patients where there is no apparent cause for the cessation of periods once the pattern has been established it is necessary to consider other reasons than physical failure. Anxiety, stress and environmental factors play a major role, so if the patient can be relieved of mental problems normal menstruation may recommence.

Dysfunctional uterine bleeding

Uterine bleeding is described as dysfunctional if it cannot be associated with normal menstruation and has no apparent traumatic cause. It may be irregular in time (metrorrhagia) or excessive in amount (menorrhagia). If pelvic diseases are excluded dysfunctional uterine bleeding can often be attributed to an endocrine disorder. One reason, particularly in young women, is due to failure of ovulation ie anovular bleeding. In the absence of a corpus luteum the secretion of progesterone is suppressed causing a prolonged regeneration of the endometrium. The resulting condition is known as metropathia haemorrhagia. The main symptom is an irregular period every six to eight weeks with excessive bleeding resulting from the massive proliferation of the endometrium.

Treatment

The patient will be admitted to hospital for investigation to confirm the diagnosis. A curettage is performed to remove minute sections of the endometrium for laboratory examination. To enable the curette to pass into the uterus safely the cervix must be dilated, which is why the operation is known as dilatation and curettage (D and C). It is considered minor surgery in that no incisions are made in the abdomen or vagina but the nurse must remember that the patient still incurs surgical trauma and is subject to many of the major post-operative problems.

The patient is admitted the day before operation for preparation including a bath, signing the consent form and premedication. On return from theatre she will be observed for haemorrhage. The perineal dressing should be inspected at intervals and a record of the patient's pulse and blood pressure is made to indicate undetected haemorrhage. The patient may complain of low back pain caused by the position on the operating table but this usually passes within a short while, although mild analgesics may be necessary if the pain persists. She will get up on the following day and be discharged home if satisfactory.

Hormone therapy for dysfunctional uterine bleeding encourages the natural formation of the corpus luteum. Progesterone can be given daily either as a short-term measure in an attempt to induce a normal cycle or as a continuous replacement therapy. Oral contraceptive agents may be prescribed also to create a normal menstrual cycle.

Hormone treatment is not always satisfactory and in some cases hysterectomy is the most suitable alternative. Hysterectomy is removal of the uterus and it may be performed through the vagina or through an abdominal incision.

Neoplasms and cysts

The ovary is subject to the development of cysts and tumours, of these one group produce hormones and are classified as functional tumours. Many of them are rare including arrhenoblastoma, theca cell and luteoma and are not described here. One is more frequently seen, called granulosa cell tumour.

Granulosa cell tumour

This tumour is composed of cells similar to those of the Graafian follicle and causes a rise in the level of oestradiol. It is malignant and can affect women of any age although the majority of patients are over the age of forty years. The effect is dependent on the age of the patient. In children it will cause precocious puberty and early development of secondary sex characteristics. In young girls it will produce a mature uterus and periodic bleeding. In women of reproductive age it causes changes in the menstrual cycle such as menorrhagia or amenorrhoea. In post menopausal women where normal ovarian secretions are minimal it will have a refeminising effect causing cyclical bleeding to start again. Because of its malignancy this tumour is removed surgically.

Hormonal theories of dysmenorrhoea and pre-menstrual tension

Dysmenorrhoea is a term used to describe menstruation that is so painful that it incapacitates the sufferer. It is thought to be caused by an imbalance of ovarian hormones in a woman who otherwise has normal ovulatory cycles. This theory is strengthened by the fact that women with anovulatory cycles do not suffer with dysmenorrhoea. In severe cases treatment is directed at inhibiting ovulation by the administration of oestrogens. Patients complain of severe abdominal colic, backache and nausea. Analgesics such as paracetemol are effective in many cases.

Pre-menstrual tension describes a variety of symptoms experienced by women immediately before menstruation, including headache, depression, abdominal discomfort, mastalgia and nervousness. Some symptoms may be psychological in origin while others are due to excessive secretion of oestrogens. There is often a retention of body water and the onset of the symptoms may be preceded by a low urinary output and an increase in weight. Progesterone during the latter half of the cycle can be effective in reducing the symptoms.

Therapeutic use of ovarian hormones

Progesterone

Although progesterone is naturally produced it can also be made synthetically. It has a number of therapeutic uses in addition to those already mentioned.

Endometriosis

This is a condition in which the endometrium grows in sites other than the lining of the uterus. It can cause ovarian cysts or in extreme circumstances spread to other pelvic organs. Progesterone may be given to depress the excessive growth of endometrium.

Infertility

Infertility is a compound problem. If no physical defects are found to prevent conception, failure to ovulate may be the cause. In all cases however a woman is unlikely to become pregnant if her progesterone secretion is insufficient for this stops the correct development of the endometrium. Progesterone may be given during the latter half of the cycle.

Abortion
Threatened and habitual abortion can result from low levels of progesterone being secreted before the placenta is able to secrete its hormones. Progesterone may be given during the first months of pregnancy to overcome this lack.

Oestrogen
Synthetic oestrogens are widely used and include stilboestrol which was the first and is the most potent of the group.

Climacteric symptoms
Oestrogen can relieve the symptoms associated with the menopause, particularly when induced by surgery. The menopause involves a high degree of psychological stress related to the loss of reproductive function and anticipated loss of libido. The nervous system is subject to vasomotor upsets causing 'hot flushes', emotional irritability, depression and lack of concentration are also associated. In cases where the symptoms are pronounced oestrogens may be given with reduction of the dosage slowly as the body readjusts to the change.

Post menopausal atrophic conditions
After the menopause ovulation ceases and the hormones necessary for reproduction are greatly reduced. Oestrogens affect the mucous membrane of the vagina by creating a protective environment against bacteria. When oestrogen secretion ceases the vagina atrophies and is more prone to inflammatory conditions. Stilboestrol can be given orally for two to three weeks to reduce these symptoms.

Suppression of lactation
Lactation is partly initiated by low oestrogen levels at parturition. When lactation needs to be suppressed stilboestrol is prescribed to prevent painful breast engorgement.

9

The Breast

When diseases of the breast are mentioned women immediately think of cancer. The fear of cancer, in all its forms, is deeply rooted in the minds of most people. Great efforts have been made through radio, television and the press to counteract this fear by spreading accurate information. Early detection of cancer offers the best chance of successful treatment and this is particularly relevant to cancer of the breast. As more is known about the diagnosis and treatment of cancer greater numbers of patients are asking for information and advice, and it is often to nurses that such patients look for help. This applies to all nurses whether working in the community, industry or in hospital wards and departments. In their daily contact with patients they have an unrivalled opportunity to assist in overcoming this widespread fear and to encourage women to make use of such measures as cervical smear tests and regular examination of their breasts.

The breast is not an endocrine gland and does not secrete hormones, but it merits a chapter in this book because of its close relationship to the ovary and pituitary gland both in development and function. Nurses should be familiar with the structure and function of the breast, or mammary gland, because of the important pathology associated with it.

The two female mammary glands are specialised organs that develop in the tissues of the thoracic wall. Development begins at the age of puberty, eleven to fourteen years, and up to this time the nipple is the only visible indication of breast tissue. The breast is composed of fifteen to twenty lobes of glandular tissue similar to that forming the sweat glands, they are arranged around the nipple in a radial pattern. Between each glandular lobe are bands of connective tissue holding them in position, these are interspaced with adipose tissue particularly in the surface areas. Leading from the glandular ducts are tiny sacs or alveoli, their size and number fluctuate according to the hormonal influence affecting them at any specific time.

The blood supply of the breast is derived from branches of the mammary, lateral thoracic and intercostal arteries. The venous return is

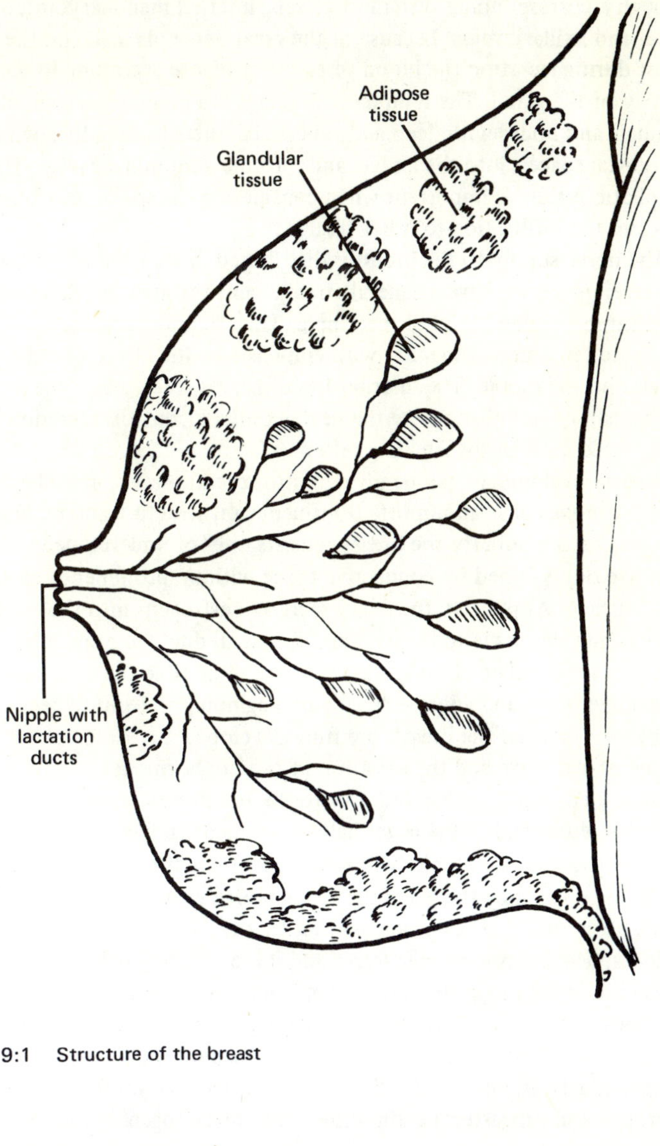

Fig 9:1 Structure of the breast

through a corresponding system of vessels, internal mammary, intercostal and axillary veins. Because of the great demands made on the breast during lactation the blood vessels vary in size according to the activity of the gland. The lymphatic drainage is a complex system of channels and nodes with deep and superficial ducts leading through the intercostal spaces, into the axillae and into the abdominal cavity. The lymphatic system is important when considering the spread of malignant cells and the infiltration to other tissues.

The nerve supply to the breast is distributed in a particular pattern. The afferent nerves have a general arrangement through the gland with large numbers in and around the nipple. The efferent nerves are distributed in a similar manner with emphasis on the ducts, blood vessels and the nipple. The distribution of nerves is related to the mechanism of lactation where the nerve complex controls secretion of breast milk through the suckling reflex.

Breast development can be divided into several phases, in each of these hormones have an important influence on structure and secretory changes. Before puberty the breast consists only of undeveloped primitive ducts joined by connective tissue with no prominence on the body surface. At puberty the ovary secretes oestrogens into the circulation causing the tissue to increase and the small ducts to grow into glandular lobes called alveolar ducts. At the same time the supporting connective fibres and adipose tissues are beginning to form. When maturity is reached the breasts are fully developed due to the effect of the menstrual cycle and the variation of ovarian hormones to which the glands are constantly subjected. Oestrogen and progesterone directly affect the ducts and in the latter half of the menstrual cycle congestion and sensitivity of the nipples will precede menstruation.

During pregnancy the glandular tissue increases under the influence of the hormonal changes produced first by the ovaries and then by the placenta. The breasts become larger and more sensitive being engorged by the increased blood supply, the tension can be so great as to cause striations of the skin. During the second half of pregnancy a yellow, watery fluid called colostrum may be expressed by the breast consisting of water, fatty globules and cell debris. After parturition the level of oestrogen and progesterone diminishes and the lactogenic factor is

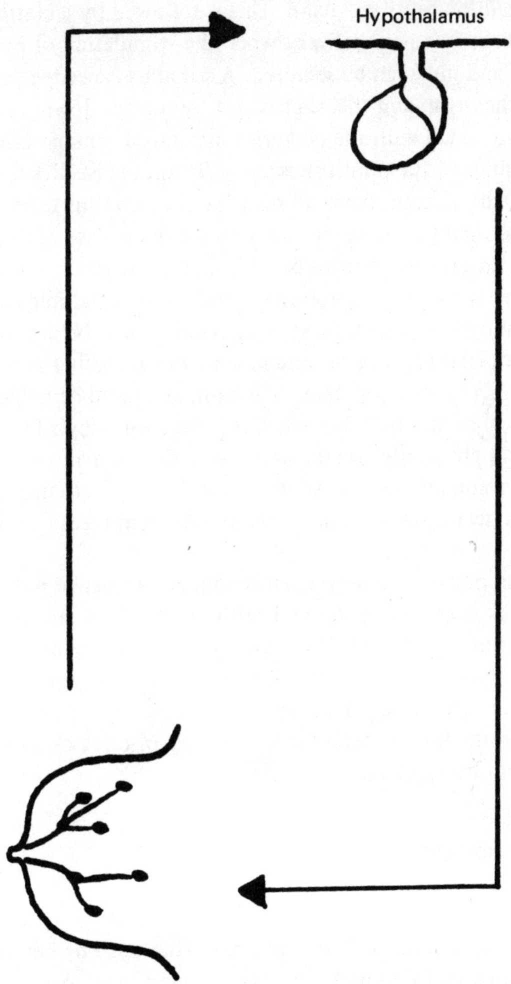

Fig 9:2 The 'let down' reflex

released from the pituitary gland. This is followed by lactation on the third or fourth day after delivery when the stimulation of prolactin is unopposed and milk can be secreted. A stimulus is needed for milk to pass from the organ and this is provided by the 'let down' reflex, a complex associated with the posterior pituitary hormone oxytocin. The simple stimulus of the infant sucking at the nipple is sufficient to create impulses in the afferent nerve fibres which are transmitted to the pituitary via the hypothalamus. This causes the release of oxytocin which stimulates the expression of milk. This delicate reaction is easily disturbed particularly by emotional stress. Nurses and midwives should encourage mothers to look forward to feeding their babies, to regard it as a time of pleasure, comfort and ease in which mother and child take delight in each other's company. The mother should be helped to plan her routine in such a way that when it is time for baby's feed she is mentally and physically relaxed and distractions are at a minimum. Anxiety, tension and fatigue are the main factors that inhibit the flow of milk in a healthy mother and prevent her from feeding her child.

Lactation normally ceases when the infant is weaned but certain conditions such as poor maternal health or still birth can demand that lactation is not established. The secretion of milk may be prevented by the administration of oestrogen. Stilboestrol is usually used for one to two weeks in daily doses of 10mg.

Although the breast is subject to a variety of diseases they are best considered in two groups.

1 Tumours
2 Inflammation

Tumours

The breast is a common site for tumours. They may be benign or malignant. Benign tumours are generally found in women up to the age of thirty-five years, and are easily removed. Tumours after this age may be malignant and they are responsible for a large number of deaths each year.

Benign tumours

The common type of benign tumour found in the breast is called a fibro-adenoma which is a growth of glandular and fibrous tissues. The patient may complain that her periods are irregular and that she suffers from varying degrees of discomfort each month before she menstruates. She may also find the lump in the breast grows bigger when she is menstruating. Like benign tumours in other parts of the body the growth is encapsulated and is usually mobile when palpated. It is not unusual to find more than one tumour at the same time and as many as four or five may develop together in the same region of the breast. Although at this time the growth is not malignant it is considered advisable to remove it surgically as there could be malignant changes if left untreated. Treatment requires a short stay in hospital where the growth is removed and sent to the laboratory for tests to ensure that no malignancy is present. The patient will need to return to have the skin sutures removed a few days later.

Patients tend to ask nurses questions about their health when in hospital and one question is about the method of self examination of the breast for unfamiliar lumps. This examination should be carried out each month, it does not take long and the relief from worry is a satisfactory reward. It has been recommended that this examination should start from about the age of twenty years and continue through life. It is best performed a few days after menstruation when the breasts are not engorged and the tissues are loose and palpable. It will also ensure that the examination is carried out regularly.

Self examination

It is important to appreciate that all breast tumours are not painful and may give no pain even when located and touched. Because of this a woman may consider that a lump is of no importance and ignore it whilst still being aware of its presence.

Self examination does not take more than a few minutes, the only requirements are a large towel and a mirror. As it is necessary to lie down for part of the test it is best conducted in the bedroom.

The woman should undress to the waist and stand in a good light in front of a mirror. This part of the test is concerned with visual changes and should begin with the arms hanging at the sides. First the shape of both breasts is noted for the differences between them. Other observations include puckering of the skin, rashes, retraction of the nipple and discharges or bleeding from the nipple. Any changes should be noted. The procedure is then repeated turning first to one side and then the other. This is important as some differences may not be detected from the front view. The process is then repeated with the arms raised above the head. The act of raising the arms causes breast tissue to change its form due to muscle and skin movement. To ensure that a constant position is adopted the hands can be clasped behind the head, this is also much less tiring than keeping the arms fully extended. Again careful visual inspection from the front followed by each side is necessary.

The second part of the examination requires the subject to lie on the bed. This allows the natural 'flow' of breast tissue across the chest wall. The towel is folded and placed under the left ribs raising the left side of the chest, the left arm is raised and placed behind the head. This position allows a mild degree of muscle tension and offers a firmer base to examine the soft tissues on that side (photograph A).

Starting at the upper and outer quadrant of the left breast the right hand is used to palpate the deep breast tissues (photograph B). The finger should be extended the pads of the fingers being used to distinguish any changes. Gentle but firm pressure is applied with a slight rotatory movement of the hand. Moving slowly one finger's width at a time continue downward until the lower outer quadrant is reached (photograph C). If any point is thought to be abnormal repeat the exercise. Still with the arm behind the head proceed up the inner quadrant until the upper extent of the breast is reached (photograph D). Repeat this gentle pressure around the nipple in a circular pattern and visual inspection is made at this point for any discharge (photograph E).

Finally the left arm is removed and placed at the side and the fingertips of the right hand passed into the axilla where many lymphatic glands are located, any masses are noted that were not previously present (photograph F).

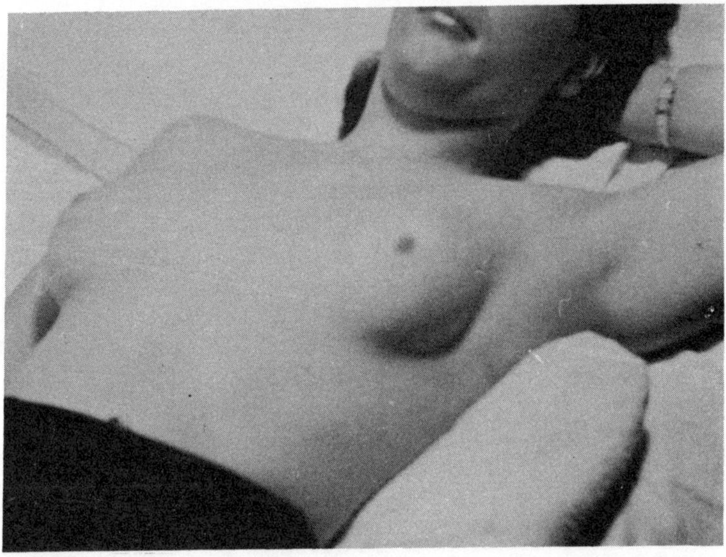
Photo A

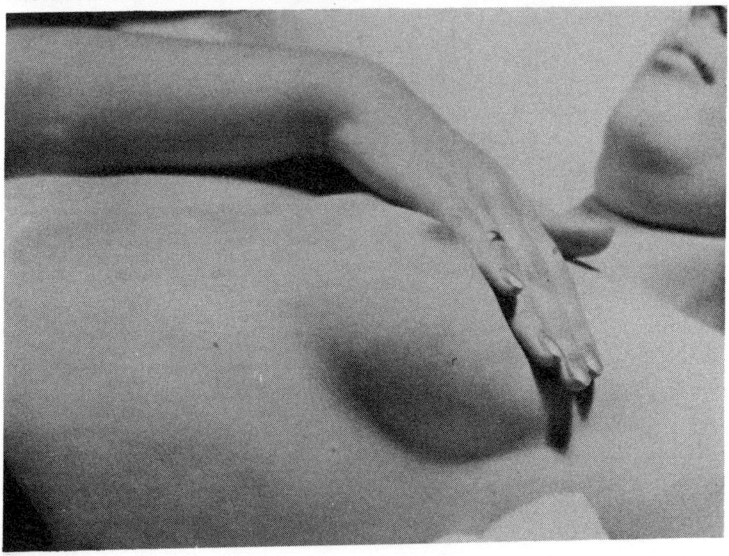
Photo B

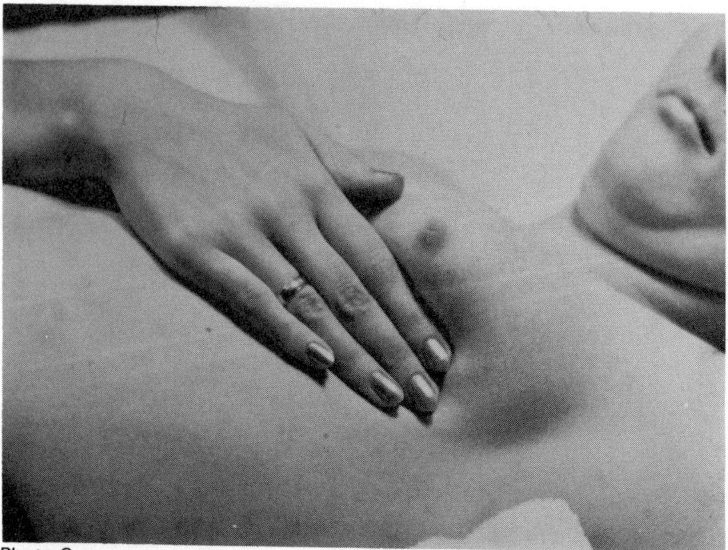

Photo C

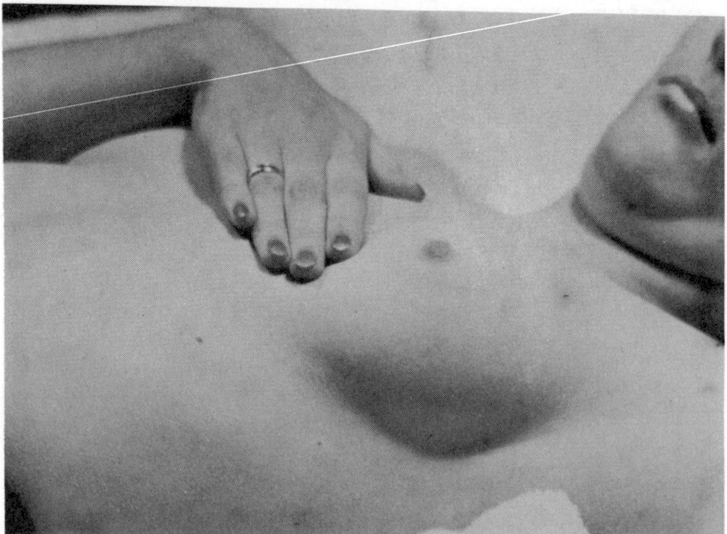

Photo D

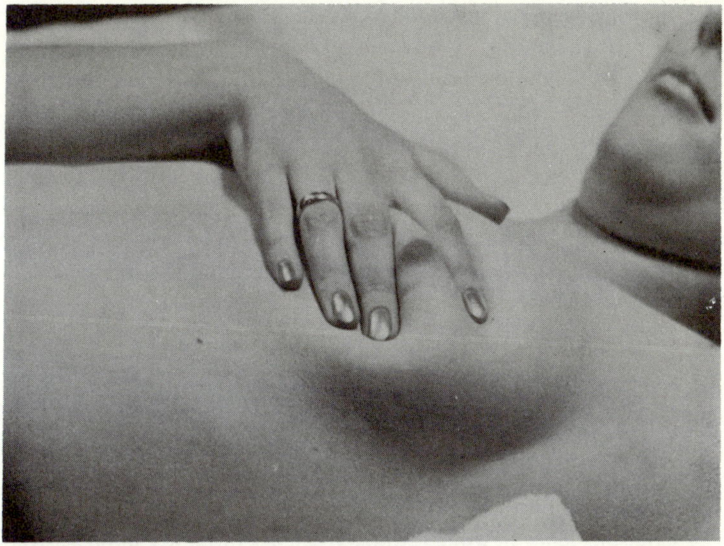
Photo E

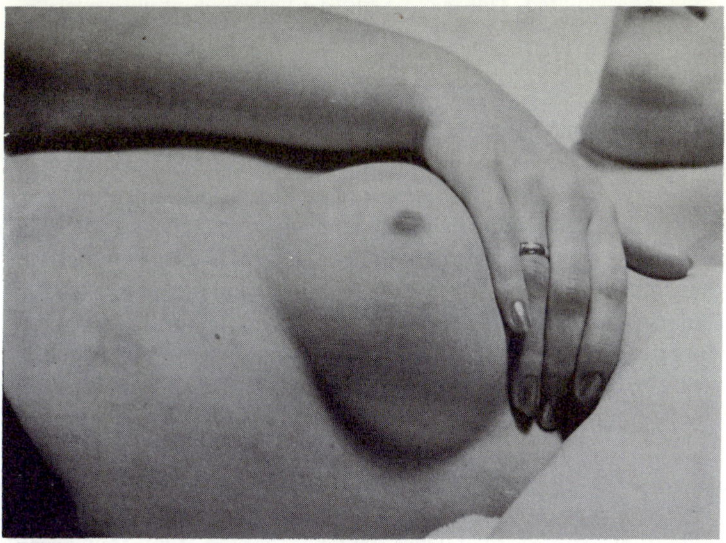
Photo F

Following examination of the axilla the procedure is completed for the left breast. The towel is now placed under the right side, the right arm is placed behind the head and the procedure is repeated using the left hand.

Malignant tumours

Malignant tumours of the breast constitute about ten to fifteen per cent. of all cancers and are most likely to be found around or after the age of the menopause. The cause of breast tumours is unknown but some contributing factors are known.

1 Hormonal influence, particularly prolonged high levels of oestrogen.

2 There is an hereditary relationship as many women with breast cancer give the history that the same disease was suffered by a parent or grandparent.

3 Although it is more common in unmarried women there is a greater incidence in women who experience difficulty in breast feeding their children. This may be another indication of hormonal influence.

Treatment

Treatment should be commenced as soon as possible. A neglected growth will increase in size and infiltrate into neighbouring structures and organs. Breast tumours can spread quicker than a similar disorder in other sites because the rich lymphatic and vascular network offers an easy passage for cells to pass from the original growth to new areas. These include the lungs, pleura, skeleton, liver and the other breast. Treatment can be by surgery, radiotherapy or hormone therapy. It is often thought best for the surgeon to remove as much of the tissue having malignant cells as he can and then any malignant cells remaining may be eliminated with radiotherapy.

Surgery

The time leading to the patient's admission has probably been a period of emotional stress for her. Once she takes the step of informing her doctor she is bound for her own safety and health to accept the sequence of care and treatment that follows. Nevertheless in finding out the diagnosis she is facing something that she has dreaded, the fear of cancer is often connected with dying and physical mutilation. The nurse can expect to receive a patient with emotional stress and anxiety when admitted to the surgical ward and she should treat her with sensitivity and consideration. In addition to this stress the patient may also be suffering with menopausal symptoms and the added change brought on by this hormonal change.

This kind of patient needs cherishing. The nurse should try to build up her confidence by every means possible. It is a good practice to allow visiting at any convenient time and the nurse's efforts to instil confidence in the patient should extend to her visitors also because their estimation of the patient's prospects will colour her outlook considerably. Privacy, courtesy and interest in the patient as an individual, which should be a part of all nursing care, are vitally important to this woman.

It is also helpful if the patient can be visited by someone who has undergone the operation and made a full recovery. Fortunately many patients who have made a full recovery themselves are pleased to offer this service since they know from personal experience what misery the patient is suffering. Such a person can discuss the problems she has encountered and the way she has adjusted to them. She can also answer questions about the special type of brassiere that the patient may wear on discharge and the patient can see for herself how reassuringly normal her visitor looks. What is most important to the patient is the knowledge that recovery is possible without any distressing after effects, and this is clear from her visitor's appearance and manner.

During the pre-operative period physiotherapy is started, particularly exercises for breathing and posture. Chest movements will be restricted immediately following the operation and early assistance to breath correctly are important. The patient's posture will be affected by the limited muscle movement on the affected side. Her carriage and stance will play an important part in her physical and psychological recovery when she is discharged.

The patient will be prepared for operation in the normal way with extra care of the skin on the affected side. Careful shaving of the axilla is necessary and cleansing of the skin should include the upper arm, the body from clavicle to umbilicus and across to the breast on the unaffected side. This preparation may frighten the patient into thinking it is a bigger operation than she anticipated but the nurse can reassure her and explain the need for care of the surrounding skin and not just the operation site.

Immediate post-operative care is partly governed by the wishes of the surgeon. Some require the patient's arm to remain at her side for the first few days to prevent undue movement over the wound while others prefer a little movement of the arm on the affected side. There will be a drain in the wound which will be observed for oozing and haemorrhage and any drainage will be recorded. Should a haematoma develop or fluid, collect it may be drained by the attachment of a mild suction apparatus such as a Redivac bottle.

An important nursing function is to assist the patient when coughing. With such vast superficial thoracic surgery pain during chest movements is inevitable and the patient will be unwilling to cough deeply. Support should be given by light pressure over the wound to prevent undue stretching and the nurse should emphasise the importance of coughing and deep breathing to reduce the risk of respiratory infection.

Two important aspects of nursing care are concerned with the patient's physical and psychological attitudes. Post-operatively the physiotherapist will commence exercises to recover movement and function. The exercises involve simple movements of the arms and the nurse should encourage the patient to practice them at regular intervals throughout the day. It is important that the patient is shown how to stand and walk correctly so that any restricted movement on the affected side can be adjusted. All these actions may be painful for the patient both physically and mentally by her unconscious wish to bend forward and hide her embarrassment. During this time she will need both assistance to stand and walk correctly and a great deal of encouragement to accept the situation in its true light – that she is not so different as she first imagined.

At first the patient will have a great difficulty in looking at the wound and the view of herself in the mirror will be a shock. The nurse should realise that adjustment takes time and should not hurry the patient but encourage her to examine the site and bathe it regularly when healing is complete. Her aim is to help the patient accept that this disfigurement need not be disabling and to care for herself when not supported by the hospital team after discharge.

Adjustment is particularly difficult for married women and the ward staff should encourage the patient to talk to her husband, to discuss the treatment she is receiving and her thoughts for the future. This is not easy for the patient and the nurse can help by making sure that the patient and her husband are given uninterrupted privacy on these occasions.

The intelligent use of a suitable prosthesis can greatly help the patient's recovery. They are extremely efficient and made of synthetic substances closely resembling breast tissue such as soft foam or a thick fluid contained in a plastic mould.

Radiotherapy

The use of radiotherapy in cancer of the breast is dependent on the degree of involvement of surrounding tissues. It may be used in combination with surgery if infiltration of the growth is deep, or as an alternative to surgery if it is localised. Either high voltage or cobalt rays are used. If radiotherapy follows surgery it is not started until healing is complete, when it is given over a period of several weeks by attendance as an outpatient. The patient may be admitted at intervals for assessment of progress.

Hormone therapy

The mammary gland is constantly subjected to circulating hormones during its development and after maturity. In some cases it is possible to restrict the growth of a tumour by variation of the hormone environment. This is mainly used as a measure for those cases in which cancer reappears after mastectomy or radiotherapy, in the elderly patient or when the disease is inoperable. Hormone changes can be brought about by surgical or medical methods. The changes depend upon the age of the patient and whether she is pre-menopausal or post-menopausal, each having a different hormone pattern. It is not expected that hormone therapy will effect a complete cure as the majority of breast cancers are advanced before this treatment is used. It is employed in order to improve the life of the patient and relieve the pain that can rise from metastases particularly in the vertebrae where pain can be intense.

Medical. Pre-menopausal women are given hormones that supress the output of natural ovarian secretions. Thus androgens are given to counter the effect of oestrogens. Post-menopausal women are given hormones to recreate the output of active ovaries. Oestrogen may be used for this purpose.

Surgical. Oophorectomy and adrenalectomy are performed to lower the level of ovarian hormones. Hypophysectomy will lower the output of gonadotrophins and stop ovarian stimulation. These operations are performed when there are widespread metastases from a breast cancer. In all cases replacement of the hormones other than ovarian secretions is necessary.

Inflammation

The common inflammatory condition affecting the breast is acute mastitis. This is usually confined to women in the early weeks of lactation and is caused by infection in the cracks around the nipple that are produced by constant moisture. It can be avoided if the nipples are bathed regularly and lanoline applied to keep the skin supple in the weeks before parturition. The condition is extremely painful and because of possible harm to the infant it is necessary for the mother to stop breast feeding and suppress lactation.

If the inflammation involves deeper tissues an abscess can form. A swinging temperature is a sign of an accumulation of pus under pressure and requires investigation. Relief of a breast abscess is achieved by incision and drainage. Specimens of pus will be sent for culture and sensitivity so that a suitable antibiotic can be given. In this condition it is imperative that breast feeding is stopped immediately.

Nursing care of this patient is directed towards the relief of pain by giving adequate support for the breast with a firm many tailed bandage. The patient needs as much rest as possible as she may be exhausted due to the recent combination of pain and lactation. Mild analgesics such as

Paracetemol are given. If lactation is to be stopped the fluid intake is restricted. Excess milk is withdrawn, not by squeezing but with a breast pump as direct pressure on the breast can cause the infection to spread. To reduce chances of further filling the breasts are bound with a wide crepe bandage because they have sufficient elasticity for movement while maintaining firm pressure. To aid the suppression of lactation the patient is given stilboestrol.

10
Oral Contraceptives

Oral contraceptive agents are physiologically related to hormones and their effect on body function. Although not a topic directly related to nurses or nursing it is included to enlighten the reader in the uses and problems of this much discussed drug group. The controlled use of these agents has a place in the world today where an ever-increasing population is continually creating fresh economic difficulties, particularly in the developing countries who are striving to attain a stable way of life. Even in Britain the advent of oral contraceptives has resulted in a new approach to family planning at government level through the introduction of the National Health Service (Family Planning Act) 1967 allowing Local Health Authorities throughout the country to open clinics, offer free advice and give assistance to the community on family planning matters.

Before the introduction of oral contraceptives the effectiveness of other conventional contraceptive techniques left much to be desired. Failure rates were consistently high until the introduction of the intrauterine contraceptive device (IUDC). Even here failures are found due to unobserved expulsion of the device from its position in the uterus. Following the introduction of 'the pill' the number of people practising organised family planning has risen considerably. Among the many advantages offered by oral contraception over other conventional methods are the ease and simplicity of use and removal of the aesthetically disturbing effect of mechanical methods. There are however a number of women who are unable to use oral contraceptive agents due to physical contra-indications. Allowance must also be made for one's religious and moral beliefs when considering the use of these drugs.

Pharmacology

For many years it had been known that the hormones oestrogen and progestogen can be used to suppress ovulation. Full use of this knowledge was not possible until the discovery of synthetic hormones that could be taken by mouth and still remain active. The first successful breakthrough was about 1965 and since this time a number of pharmaceutical companies have devoted much time and research to improve the quality and safety of these drugs, stimulated by the vast potential market throughout the world. The result of this work is shown by the effectiveness of the products available today.

One major problem of the oral contraceptive group is the risk of complications developing including deep vein thrombosis and pulmonary embolism. Complications have a direct relationship with the quantity of oestrogen in each tablet. Although the mortality figures are extremely low the government appointed a committee to evaluate the hazards and find means of avoiding them. This safety committee found that high oestrogen levels are liable to precipitate complications in susceptible women. They recommended 50 micrograms as the maximum oestrogen content of each tablet. Progestogens were found not to be contributing factors.

Oral contraceptive agents are divided into two main groups. Those containing a combination of oestrogen and progestogen sometimes called the 'Pinctus pill' after one of the men associated with its development. The other provides oestrogen during the first part of the cycle followed by a combination of oestrogen and progestogen, these are called 'sequential pills'. Because they are artificially produced synthetic hormones have different names to natural ovarian hormones.

OESTROGENS	PROGESTOGENS
Ethinyloestradiol	Norethisterone
Mestranol	Megestrol acetate
	Chlormadinone acetate

Action and efficiency

It is not certain how the drug affects natural reproductive function. It has been found that ovulation is suppressed by the administration of drugs in this group. In those women where ovulation continued other changes occur to make the chance of pregnancy difficult; changes in the endometrium or increased viscosity of cervical mucous are examples of these. The efficiency of these drugs is beyond question. During tests and trials over a number of years the failure rate is negligible. Even when unintended pregnancies have occurred they can frequently be attributed to forgotten tablets, stopping of tablets for short periods of hospitalisation, ignorance, misunderstanding of the instructions and financial difficulties preventing the purchase of further supplies. Added to the efficiency of these drugs can be considered the ability to become pregnant when desired. Once the drug is discontinued chances of pregnancy taking place are not altered. Risks of multiple pregnancies are no greater than at any other time.

Side effects

Emphasis has been given to the problems of side effects. Some are produced as a direct action on body function while a large number of miscellaneous symptoms have no direct association.

Nausea
A common complaint that is responsible for many women stopping the drug.

Breakthrough bleeding
This includes 'spotting' or slight bleeding, it can occur at irregular intervals and frequently stops following several months of consecutive use.

Breast tenderness
Mastalgia is often associated with contraceptive agents particularly at the end of a menstrual cycle. This same pain is found in women not taking the drug (pre-menstrual tension) although it is increased and over a longer period of time.

Weight changes
An increase in weight is a common side effect and can be attributed to mild retention of fluid or an increase in appetite.

Rare instances of disturbance of the nervous system are found including dizziness, headache and occasional mild depression. Women of a nervous disposition may find an increase in tension developing.

Stress has been placed on the toxic effects that can result in more serious consequences. It is quite correct to consider the long term effects of these drugs as it should be with any prescribed medication. There are a number of disorders that contraindicate the use of oral contraceptives including previous liver damage, diabetes mellitus, carcinoma of the breast and any thrombo-embolic condition. Such danger can be avoided by careful examination and history before the drugs are prescribed.

Oral contraceptive drugs are designed to be taken once daily during prescribed times through the menstrual cycle, the timing is important to prevent ovulation taking place. Some products commence tablet one about the third or fourth day of the cycle counting the first day of bleeding as day one. One tablet is taken each day until twenty-one days have passed, this is followed by seven days without tablets during which withdrawal bleeding occurs. One product includes seven lactose tablets which are quite harmless but allow the patient to take one tablet daily without a break and thereby reduce the chance of mistakes.

Although primarily designed for contraceptive purposes they are also used in gynaecological disorders; particularly conditions related to menstruation, including, excessive menstrual loss (menorrhagia), painful menstruation (dysmenorrhoea), and pre-menstrual tension.

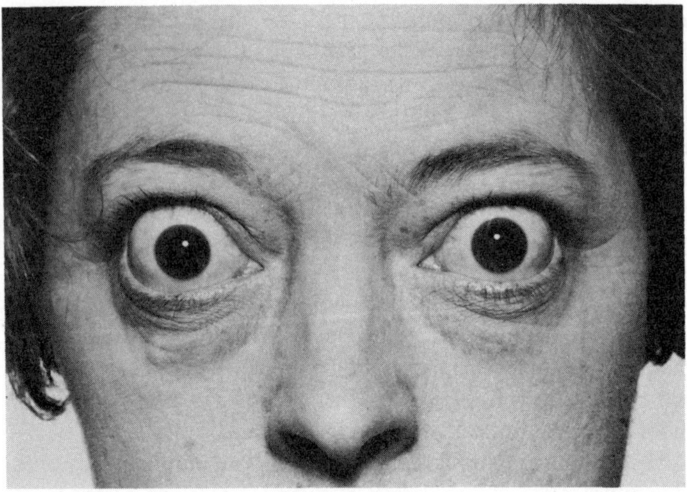

'Exophthalmos'

THYROTOXICOSIS

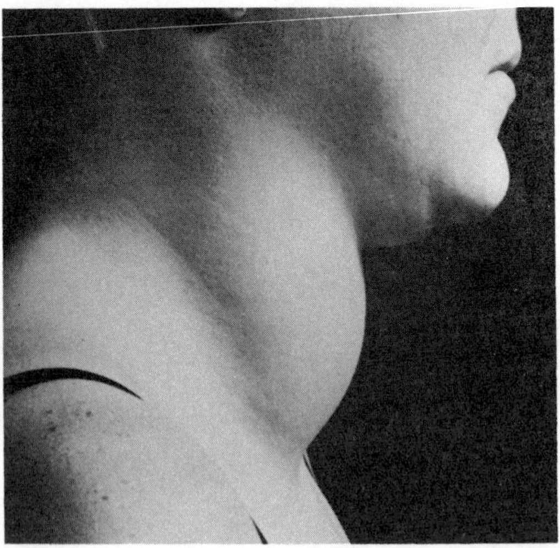

'Goitre'

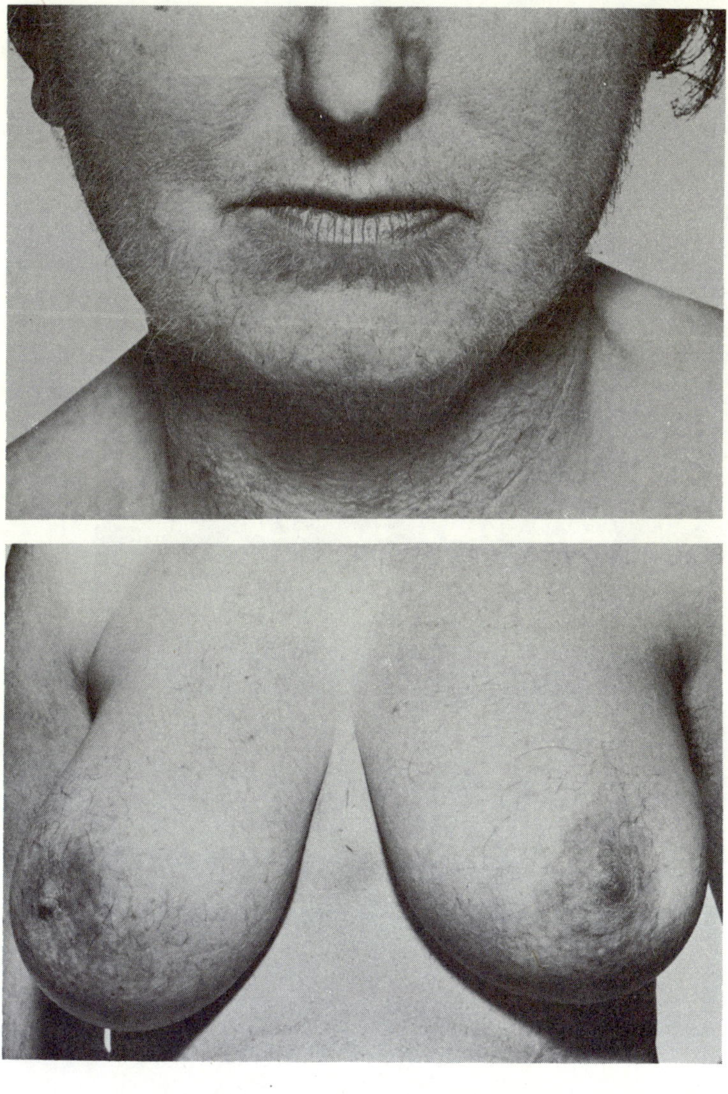

VIRILISING Tumour of the Adrenal Cortex

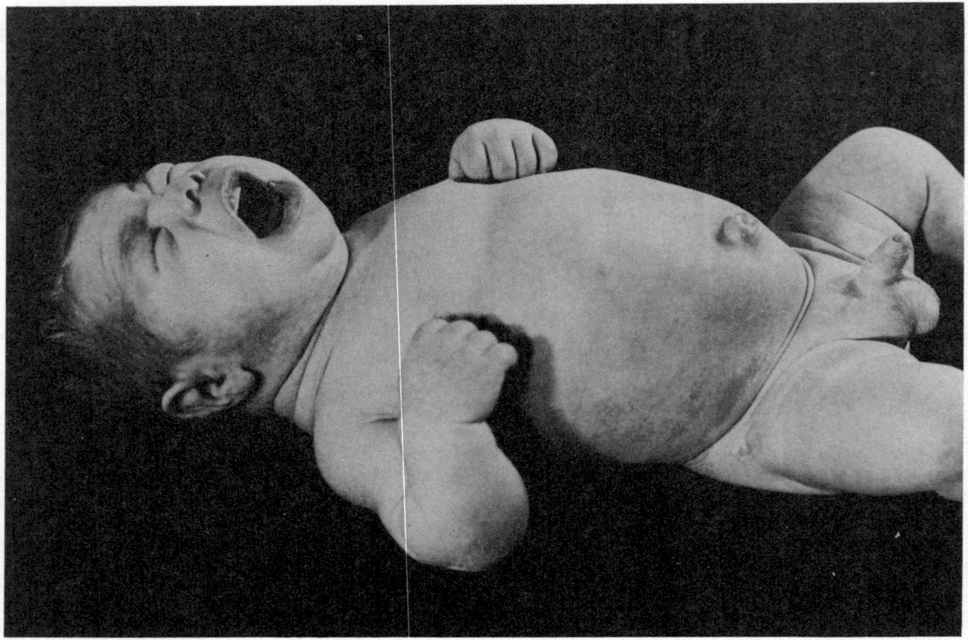

CRETINISM Before treatment

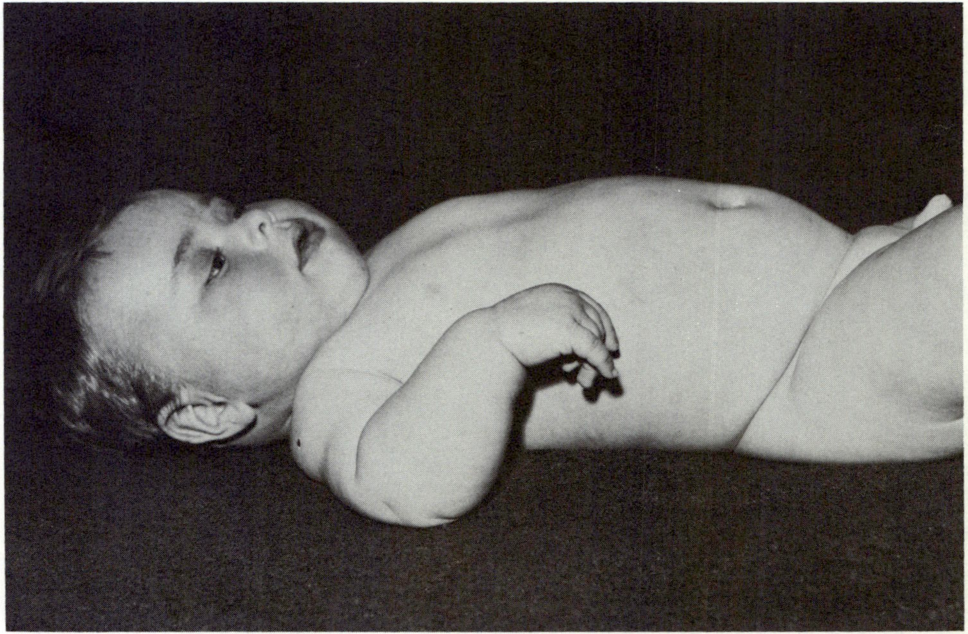

CRETINISM After treatment

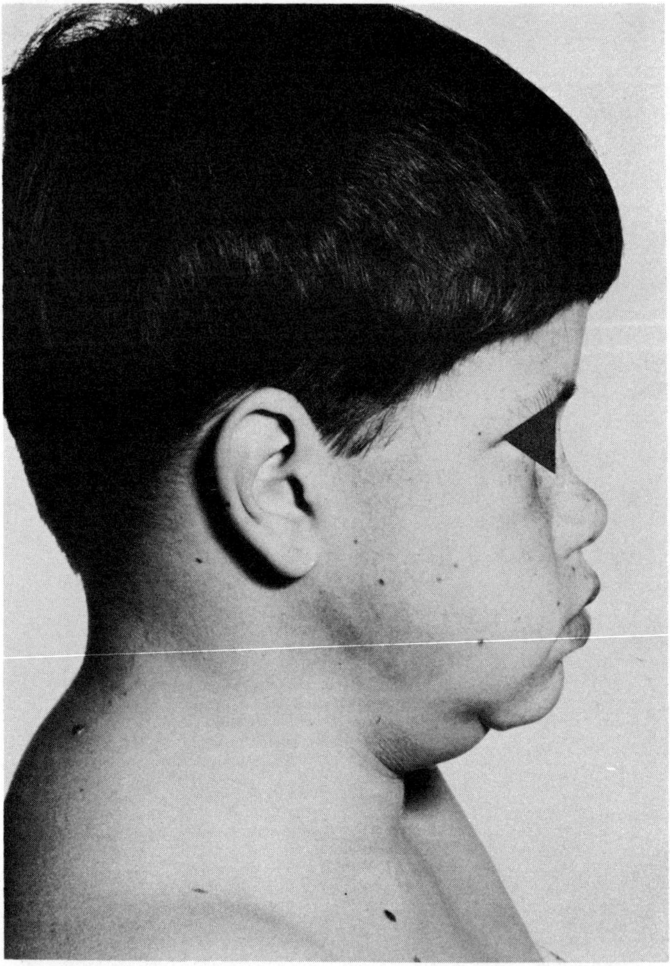

MYXOEDEMA A Before treatment

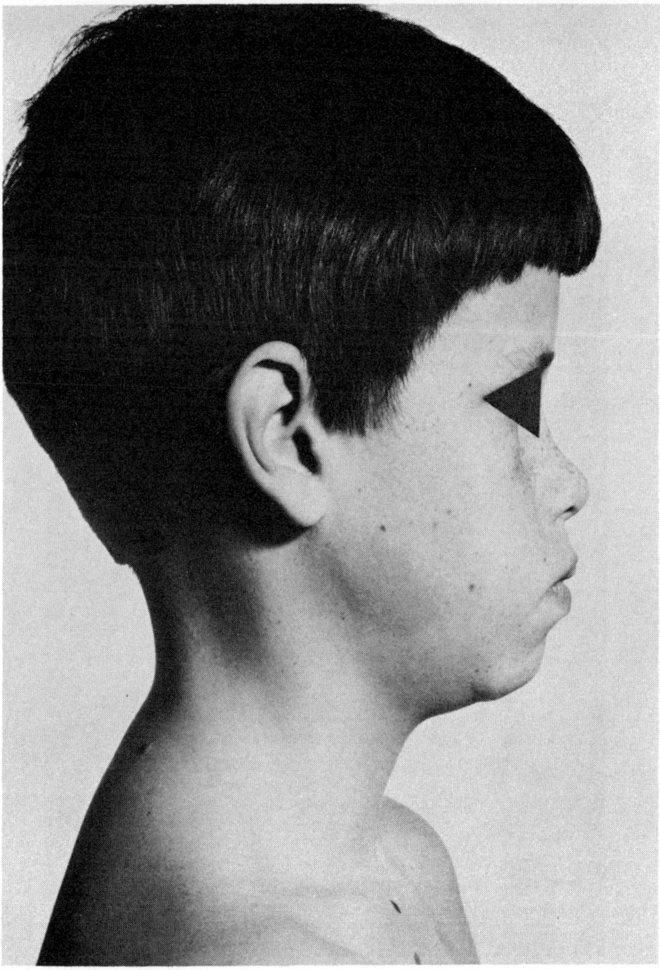

MYXOEDEMA

B After treatment

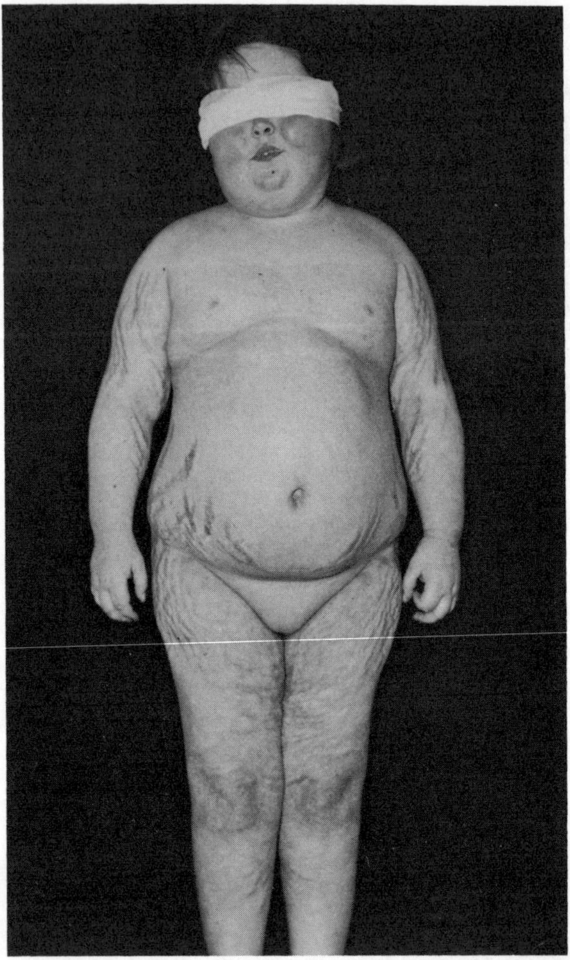

CUSHING'S SYNDROME

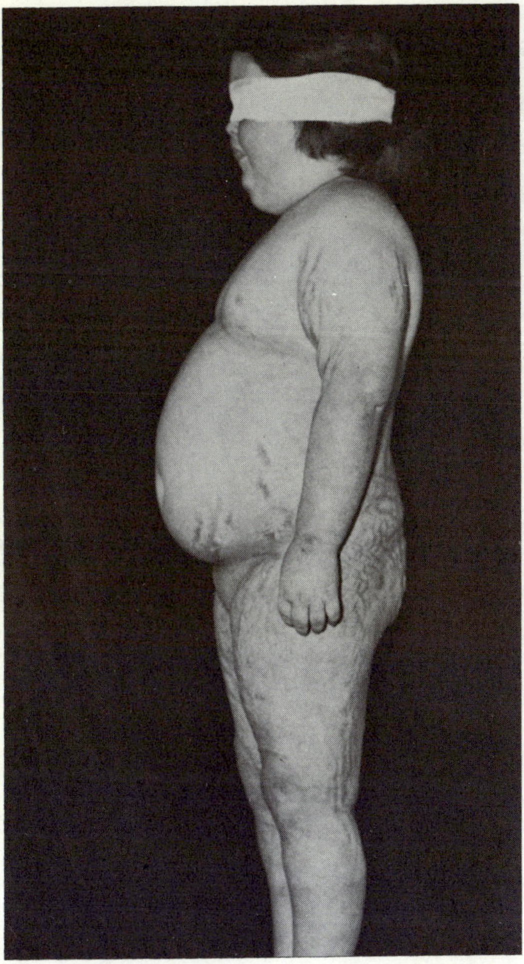

CUSHING'S SYNDROME

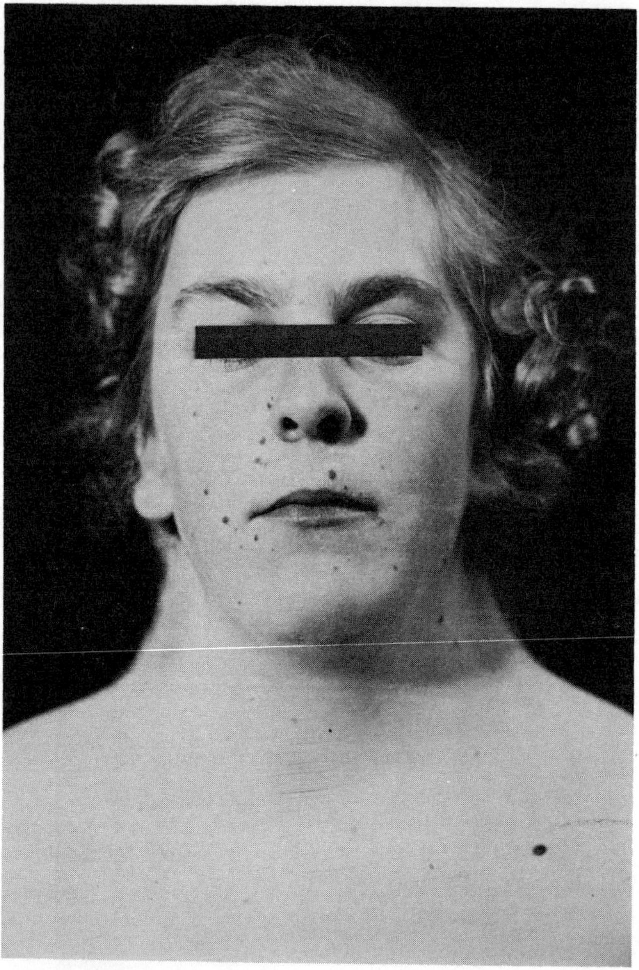

TURNER'S SYNDROME

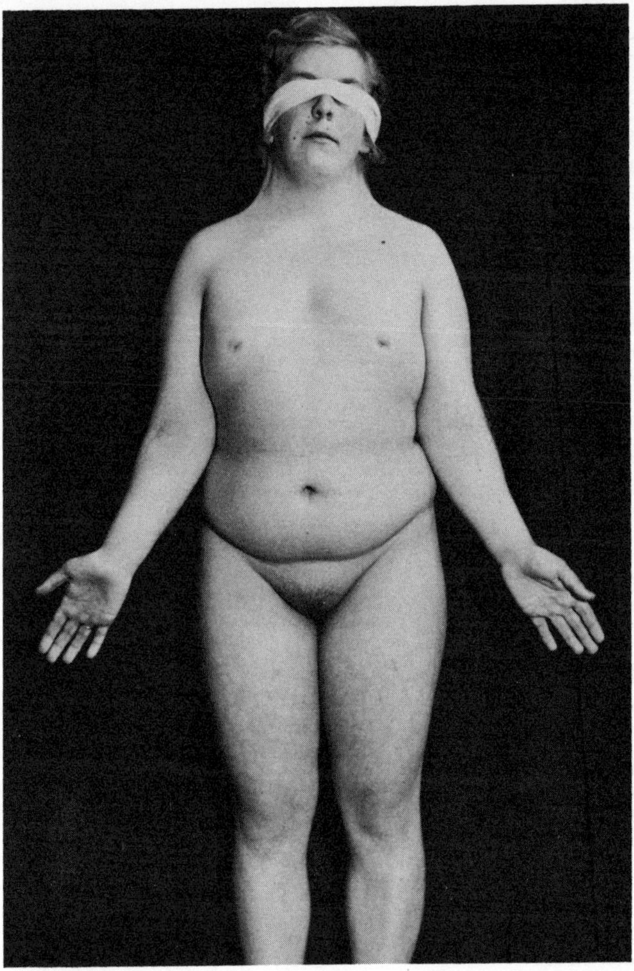

TURNER'S SYNDROME

Index